# Advances in Electroencephalography and Brain Connectome

*Edited by Tak Lap Poon*

Published in London, United Kingdom

Advances in Electroencephalography and Brain Connectome
http://dx.doi.org/10.5772/intechopen.104301
Edited by Tak Lap Poon

Contributors
Ahmad Tamimi, Iskandar Tamimi, Malik Juweid, Sergey Alexander Gulyaev, Ming-Him Yuen, Germaine Hiu-Fai Chan, Cheng King Fai Kevin, Lau Sau Ning Sarah, Grace Ho, Ting Hin Adrian Hui, See Ka Wing Michael



First published in London, United Kingdom, 2023 by IntechOpen
IntechOpen is the global imprint of INTECHOPEN LIMITED, registered in England and Wales, registration number: 11086078, 5 Princes Gate Court, London, SW7 2QJ, United Kingdom

British Library Cataloguing-in-Publication Data
A catalogue record for this book is available from the British Library

Additional hard and PDF copies can be obtained from orders@intechopen.com

Advances in Electroencephalography and Brain Connectome
Edited by Tak Lap Poon
p. cm.
Print ISBN 978-1-83768-822-7
Online ISBN 978-1-83768-823-4
eBook (PDF) ISBN 978-1-83768-824-1

# Meet the editor

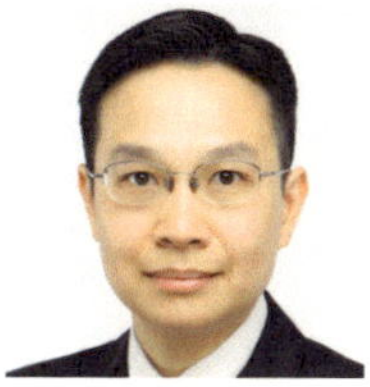

Tak Lap Poon graduated from the medical school of the University of Hong Kong in 1998. He completed neurosurgery training in 2006 and became a neurosurgical specialist. In 2006, he studied epilepsy surgery and stereotactic and functional neurosurgery in London with Mr. William Harkness from the Great Ormond Street Hospital and Mr. Andrew McEvoy from the National Hospital for Neurology and Neurosurgery. Dr. Poon currently works at Queen Elizabeth Hospital, Hong Kong, where he is the coordinator of neurosurgical services including stereotactic and functional neurosurgery, epilepsy surgery, movement disorder, stereotactic radiosurgery, and endovascular surgery. His interests include movement disorder surgery, epilepsy surgery, awake craniotomy, stereotactic and functional neurosurgery, and stereotactic radiosurgery. Dr. Poon is the president of the Hong Kong Epilepsy Society, a council member of the Hong Kong Movement Disorder Society, and a board member of the executive committee of the Asian-Australasian Society for Stereotactic and Functional Neurosurgery.

# Contents

# Preface

The study of the human brain and its functioning is an interesting and fascinating subject. Electroencephalography (EEG) and brain connectome analysis are evolving fields for understanding brain electrophysiology and its complex and interconnecting cerebral network.

EEG has been used for decades, from basic investigations in epilepsy patients to advanced studies of the propagation of pathological seizure in refractory epilepsy. The advances in the study of the brain connectome by anatomical and neuroradiological aspects supplement the mechanisms underlying cognition, behavior, and disease.

*Advances in Electroencephalography and Brain Connectome* presents a comprehensive overview of the basic principles and concepts as well as the latest developments in this field. The chapters cover a wide range of topics including laboratory practical use of EEG, EEG with correlation of neuroimaging, medical application of EEG, and connectome concepts in surgical intervention including newly evolving stereotactic electroencephalography. In addition, the book discusses the popular implementation of EEG in brain–computer interfaces for neurorehabilitation.

The book serves as a platform for sharing ideas among researchers and clinicians who are interested in the study and advancement of anatomo-clinical electrophysiology networking of the human brain and its relevant functions.

**Tak Lap Poon**
Department of Neurosurgery,
Queen Elizabeth Hospital,
Hong Kong SAR, China

Chapter 1

# Practical Recommendations for Conducting an EEG Study in a Neurophysiological Laboratory

*Sergey Alexander Gulyaev*


## Abstract

The method of electroencephalography is an accurate and objective method of recording the bioelectrical activity of the brain, used both in scientific research and in clinical practice. However, achieving a high-quality result requires a lot of preparatory work. This chapter describes the technology for conducting electroencephalographic studies, their subsequent analysis, and presentation of results that are understandable to both a specialist neurophysiologist and a practicing neurologist. You will also find a description of the organization of the EEG study, the choice of scenario, functional tests, and the basics of forming a medical report. We will also consider individual issues of organizing an EEG study in people who have had a stroke, and multichannel and functional EEG studies.


**Keywords:** electroencephalography, brainmapping, organization, clinical neurophysiology, clinical practice

## 1. Introduction

Electroencephalography is an accessible method for objective diagnosis of the functional activity of the brain, widely used in modern neurology. The main reason for the modern use of electroencephalography in clinical diagnostics is the fact that there is no time delay between the level of nutrient supply to the nerve cell and changes in the total postsynaptic potential recorded using the electroencephalographic system, which is due to the absence of organelles in nerve cells that ensure the deposition of nutrients. This makes it possible to use the EEG for diagnosing brain processes with fast dynamics that are inaccessible to other technologies, in particular, fMRI. In practice, this makes it possible to observe the features of changes in cerebral hemoperfusion in the cortical regions of the cerebral hemispheres in real time. And taking into account the peculiarities of the EEG—technology to implement an economically accessible system of functional observation / control without significant risks of adverse effects on the subject.

However, the most significant issues limiting the use of EEG at present are the training of specialists who use in their daily work either primitive diagnostic technologies in the form of visualization-phenomenological analysis or controversial mathematical methods introduced into the EEG technique back in the era of analog devices, thanks to their accessibility and ease of implementation, but lacking a convincing scientific justification [1].

To understand the place of EEG in modern neurological diagnostics, these issues need to be considered in more detail. The issue of localization of the EEG signal source and its connection with brain structures were solved as early as by Penfield in the 1940s of the last century [2], using the "10-20" system of electrode placement on the scalp, which is still used today, which made it possible to create a triangulation model for determining the basic signal, as which W. Penfield used a focal epileptic discharge. Currently, these ideas are actively used in the photogrammetric localization system, actively promoted by Magstim Corporation (USA) [3].

But due to a lack of understanding of the need to build a triangulation model, as well as attempts to revise the technology from the standpoint of other functional methods, a significant simplification of the EEG methodology was formed and the further development of electroencephalography went in two ways: The first was the use of a routine study in outpatient practice, the purpose of which was diagnostic search and active detection of epilepsy in workers of certain specialties and industries, and the purpose of the second was to scientifically search for the relationship between functional and behavioral reactions caused by various objective factors (especially those associated with the development of intracranial volumetric formations) and changes in the general nature of the EEG signal. These studies made it possible to make a number of significant observations about the nature of slow-wave rhythmic phenomena and from the connection with processes accompanied by swelling of the nervous tissue and disorders of cerebral hemoperfusion processes; however, the lack of localization technology and the search for alternative solutions led to a loss of interest in EEG in the late 1990s of the last century, with the advent of affordable radiological diagnostic systems that made it possible to obtain a two-dimensional image understandable to most specialists, comparable to traditional anatomical drawings and postmortem examination data.

At present, the creation of systems for accurate localization of the position of EEG electrodes in space [4–6], as well as the development of the latest EEG diagnostic systems with a large number of active electrodes presented in the developments (3), has revived interest in electroencephalography as an accessible a method that makes it possible to study the processes of brain activity that have fast dynamics, which are inaccessible to systems using technologies for recording the dynamics of changes in cerebral microcirculation (MRI, near-infrared spectroscopy), and the development of software products for combining the results of a spatial representation of the EEG potential distribution on the scalp with radio imaging data methods [7] made it possible to obtain information on functional changes, comparable in accuracy to the methods of X-ray neuroimaging.

This led the International Federation of the Clinical Neurophysiology (IFCN) guidelines in 2017 to adopt official recommendations for the use of advanced lead localization systems and also recommended a gradual transition from using the "10-20" system to the "10-10" system [8]. This approach makes it possible to develop new ideas for creating a system of brain mapping (brain mapping), which allows recording various functional changes in cerebral activity in real time and making their direct connection with anatomical data [9].

The development of such systems will improve the quality of life and stroke patients and accelerate their return to an active social life, which has already been shown by a number of authors [10–12].

## 2. Registration of bioelectrical activity in a routine study

**Important!**

EEG registration begins with the procedure for checking the device for electrical safety!

Make sure that the instrument is connected to the network (control computer). Wires (especially mains power wires) do not have visible damage, which are not located near water or heat sources.

Carrying out functional stress tests may be associated with the risk of developing an epileptic seizure or other paroxysmal condition. Therefore, the specialist conducting the study must have the skills to provide resuscitation and also be able to call the resuscitation team.

### 2.1 Patient preparation

The patient comes to the study in a calm state with a clean head. Best of all, in the first half of the day, in order to avoid the consequences of psycho-emotional impact.

### 2.2 Start of the study

The patient is connected using an electrode interface (cap). It is necessary to make sure that the cap is clean and dry, and the helmet material and wires do not have visible damage.

Installation of electrodes is carried out by means of the international layout of electrodes "10-20."

Installation of reference (ear) electrodes is carried out on the earlobes A1—left lobe and A2—right lobe using electrodes—clothespins.

If it is impossible to install ear electrodes (there are no clothespins in the packing or otherwise), reference electrodes are installed on the mastoid processes A1—left mastoid process and A2—right mastoid process.

After connecting the patient to the device, the photostimulator is installed at a distance of 20 cm from the eyes and the direction of the light flux is checked.

### 2.3 Next, we move on to working with the program

1. Fill out the patient card

    We enter data into the card, including full name, age, and gender

2. Checking the installation of the current installation

Most often, the current editing of the recording is set automatically, but before examining, you need to make sure that the program settings have not changed.

3. Check the write speed

    Write speed should be set to 30 mm per 1 second

4. Checking the amplitude sweep

Amplitude sweep set to 7 μV

5. Checking the settings of filtering values

The low-frequency limit is set to 0.5 Hz

The high end is set to 35 for normal exploration and 70 for advanced.

After checking the recording parameters, we start monitoring—a mode in which the device is turned on, but no data are written to the disk.

In monitoring mode, we check the characteristics of the curves and proceed to the impedance test.

6. Impedance test

The subelectrode resistance (impedance) shows the correct installation of the electrode and characterizes the contact of the electrode with the scalp. The impedance value must not exceed 10 kOm. At high impedance values, it is necessary to check the contact of the electrodes with the scalp, if necessary, remove the hair that has fallen under the electrode, add an electrically conductive gel, or thoroughly degrease the skin with an alcohol-containing solution and a cotton swab.

After stabilization of the impedance values (should be equal under all electrodes), we start recording with research.

7. Study recording

The study recording mode differs from monitoring in that the data are saved to the computer's hard drive. Recording is the main survey mode!

During the study, the patient is presented with various functional tests, which, for ease of understanding, are combined into a single-study scenario.

## 3. Study scenario

### 3.1 General scenario

The study is carried out for at least 20 minutes and includes the following procedures:

Background recording 3–5 minutes (but not less than 3 minutes)

Opening eyes—1 min. Closing eyes—1 min.

Background recording—3 min.

Test with photostimulation (rhythmic light flashes are presented with the help of a photostimulator):

- Hz—10 sec.
    - Break 5 sec

- 2 Hz—10 sec.
    - Break 5 sec
- 3 Hz—10 sec.
    - Break 5 sec
- 4 Hz—10 sec.
    - Break 5 sec
- 5 Hz—10 sec.
    - Break 5 sec
- 25 Hz—10 sec.

Background recording—3 min.
Opening eyes—1 min. Closing eyes—1 min.
Background recording 1 min.
Hyperventilation—3 min.
Background recording—5 min.
Opening eyes—1 min. Closing eyes—1 min.
Study Termination

### 3.2 Children

In children and adolescents, it is sometimes difficult to make a full-fledged recording, according to the "10-20" system due to the small size of the head, and it is also difficult for children to remain still for a long time. At the same time, due to the functional immaturity of the structures of the child's brain, the desired phenomena manifest themselves better than in adults. Thus, an EEG study in children takes at least 15 minutes and includes the following tests:

### 3.3 Scenario "Children"

Background recording 3 min
Eye opening—1 min. Eye closing—1 minute
Background recording—1 min.
Test with photostimulation (rhythmic light flashes are presented with the help of a photostimulator)

- 1 Hz—10 sec.
    - Break 5 sec
- 2 Hz—10 sec.
    - Break 5 sec

- 3 Hz—10 sec.
    - Break 5 sec
- 4 Hz—10 sec.
    - Break 5 sec
- 5 Hz—10 sec.
    - Break 5 sec
- 25 Hz—10 sec.

Background recording—1 min.
Opening eyes—1 min. Closing eyes—1 min.
Background recording—1 min.
Hyperventilation—3 min.
Background recording—3 min.
Opening eyes—1 min. Closing eyes—1 min.
Study termination

### 3.4 Epilepsy

When the diagnosis of "Epilepsy" is established, the study is carried out for 25 minutes, but not less than 20 minutes and includes the following procedures:

### 3.5 Scenario "Epilepsy"

Background recording 5 min
Opening eyes—1 min. Closing eyes—1 min.
Background recording—3 min.
Test with photostimulation (rhythmic light flashes are presented with the help of a photostimulator)

- 1 Hz—10 sec.
    - Break 5 sec
- 2 Hz—10 sec.
    - Break 5 sec
- 3 Hz—10 sec.
    - Break 5 sec
- 4 Hz—10 sec.
    - Break 5 sec

- 5 Hz—10 sec.
    - Break 5 sec
- 25 Hz—10 sec.

Continuous photo stimulation from 1 to 50 Hz

- 40 Hz—10 sec.
    - Break 5 sec
- 30 Hz—10 sec.
    - Break 5 sec
- 20 Hz—10 sec.

Background recording—3 min.
Opening eyes—1 min. Closing eyes—1 min.
Background recording—1 min.
Hyperventilation—3 min.
Background recording—3 min.
Hyperventilation—2 min
Background recording—3 min.
Opening eyes—1 min. Closing eyes—1 min.
Background recording—3 min.
Study termination

In patients who have had a cerebral stroke, of particular interest is the reaction of the bioelectrical activity of the brain to physical activity, which occurs as a result of impaired cerebral hemoperfusion and defective functioning of the collateral blood supply system.

### 3.6 Scenario "Stroke"

Background recording (passive relaxed wakefulness with closed eyes)—3 min
Opening eyes—1 min. Closing eyes—1 min.

Test with photostimulation (rhythmic light flashes are presented with the help of a photostimulator)

- 1 Hz—10 sec.
    - Break 5 sec
- 2 Hz—10 sec.
    - Break 5 sec

- 3 Hz—10 sec.
    - Break 5 sec
- 4 Hz—10 sec.
    - Break 5 sec
- 5 Hz—10 sec.
    - Break 5 sec
- 25 Hz—10 sec.

Background recording—1 min
Opening eyes—1 min. Closing eyes—1 min.
Motion test
Squeeze—unclench the right hand—3 min
Background recording—1 min
Opening eyes—1 min. Closing eyes—1 min.
Motion test
Squeezing—unclenching the left hand—3 min
Background recording—1 min
Opening eyes—1 min. Closing eyes—1 min.
Motion test
Squeeze—unclench both hands—3 min
Background recording—1 min
Opening eyes—1 min. Closing eyes—1 min.
Test with hyperventilation
Deep breathing—3 min
Opening eyes—1 min. Closing eyes—1 min.
Background recording (passive relaxed wakefulness with closed eyes)—3 min

**Important!**

With the appearance of paroxysmal epileptiform activity, the development of a seizure, the study stops!

## 4. Conducting standard functional stress tests in the study

### 4.1 Photostimulation

Photostimulation is carried out using a special device combined with an electroencephalograph, which makes it possible to produce rhythmic light flashes at a given frequency.

The color of the flash may be white or red, depending on the design of the device. The light source can be a gas discharge lamp or high-power LEDs.

### 4.2 Contraindications for the test

Pregnancy is a relative contraindication to a photostimulation test, as there is a risk of adverse effects on the fetus in the event of an epileptic seizure.

**Important!**

**When using a photostimulator with a gas discharge lamp as a light source, never test with open eyes, due to the risk of eye damage from the powerful light flux of the gas discharge lamp!!!**

### 4.3 Hyperventilation

During hyperventilation, the subject takes a deep breath (trying to fill the lungs as best as possible and exhale through slightly closed lips).

### 4.4 Contraindications for the test

Relative contraindications to the hyperventilation test:

History of indications of cardiac arrhythmias
Intracranial tumors of subtentorial localization
Myocardial infarction
Diabetes mellitus in the stage of decompensation
Acute intoxications
Chronic obstructive pulmonary disease
Frequent series of generalized and secondary generalized seizures

### 4.5 Absolute contraindications

Trauma to the upper respiratory tract
Paroxysmal ventricular arrhythmias
Acute period of myocardial infarction
Pneumothorax

In addition to the contraindications listed above, the hyperventilation test should not be continued if true epileptiform activity is clearly presented in the record, since the main goal of the test has been achieved, and its continuation may lead to the development of a clinical seizure, or in an unfavorable case, status epilepticus.

**Important!**

When performing the test, frequent, shallow, and ineffective breathing should be avoided, since in this case, the state of hyperoxia is not achieved and the test becomes ineffective.

**Important!**

The main task of a routine examination is to ESTABLISH A DIRECT RELATIONSHIP between the development of a functional disorder and the type of functional load imposed, which is confirmed by the development of pathological activity in the EEG recording!!!

In the absence of a direct connection between the development of a functional disorder and a provoking factor, it is concluded that further examination is necessary using long-term EEG recording technologies.

## 5. Long-term EEG study

### 5.1 Continued EEG study

The purpose of the study: to identify a possible pathological response to functional loads, if there is a suspicion of the likelihood of developing a seizure, but no pathology is detected on a routine examination, but there are suspicions of the development of such.

The main objective of the study is to exclude the possibility of developing a seizure in workers of complex industries.

The study is based on repeated functional stress tests for a long time (up to 3 hours)

### 5.2 Study scenario

Background recording 5 min
Opening eyes—1 min. Closing eyes – 1 min.
Background recording—3 min.
Test with photostimulation (rhythmic light flashes are presented with the help of a photostimulator):

- 1 Hz—10 sec.
  - Break 5 sec
- 2 Hz—10 sec.
  - Break 5 sec
- 3 Hz—10 sec.
  - Break 5 sec
- 4 Hz—10 sec.
  - Break 5 sec
- 5 Hz—10 sec.
  - Break 5 sec
- 25 Hz—10 sec.

Background recording—3 min.
Opening eyes—1 min. Closing eyes—1 min.
Background recording 1 min.
Hyperventilation—3 min.
Background recording—5 min.
Opening eyes—1 min. Closing eyes—1 min.
Background recording 20 min.
Study repetition (up to 6 times)
Study Termination

**Important!**

When pathological activity appears in the record, the study is terminated as the main goal is achieved and the task is completed.

After the studies, the recording stops and the data are saved, which are transferred for analysis to the doctor, who forms the medical report.

### 5.3 VideoEEG monitoring from 4 hours (in children) to 9–12 hours in adults)

**Purpose of the study:** to evaluate changes in bioelectrical activity under conditions of a decrease in external stimuli and changes in the characteristics of the bioelectrical activity of the brain caused by a change in the phases of physiological sleep).

### 5.4 Patient preparation

The patient comes to the study in a calm state with a clean head. It is best that he does not attend work on the day of the study.

With him, the patient has pajamas or a tracksuit to change into.

Before the study, the patient is explained that he will be filmed by a video camera throughout the study and he will be in bed without a blanket.

**Important!**

The patient should not take sleeping pills for the onset of sleep, but the patient does not stop taking basic drugs (especially antiepileptic ones!)!

Conducting research

The patient is connected to the device as well as for routine examination; however, the use of electrically conductive gels is inappropriate for studies lasting more than 4 hours. When planning a long study, it is better to use a special conductive paste.

**Important!**

There is no need to require the subject to be in a state of sleep. A person can be in a state of passive relaxed wakefulness or perform normal activities. The main condition is constant video recording!

**Important!**

Functional stress tests, including opening-closing of the eyes, rhythmic photostimulation, and hyperventilation during sleep monitoring are NOT PERFORMED! Due to the possible disruption of the process of falling asleep.

All functional stress tests are carried out at the stage of a routine examination and an extended EEG examination!

**During night sleep monitoring, the following events are noted:**

1. Time of arrival of the patient in the ward

2. Bedtime

3. Light off time

4. Time of onset of sleep

5. Events (woke up, went to the toilet, etc.)

6. Main wake up time

7. Light on time

8. Time when the patient left the room.

After the studies, the recording stops and the data are saved, which are transferred for analysis to the doctor, who forms the medical report.

## 5.5 Ambulatory EEG monitoring (not always present in EEG laboratories!)

It is the longest version of the EEG—examination.

Purpose of the study: to establish how changes in the bioelectrical activity of the brain affect the daily life of the subject

The main task: to establish a direct relationship between the development of pathological bioelectrical activity and a violation of the quality of life of the subject.

Ambulatory EEG—monitoring is carried out using special mobile devices similar to ECG monitoring devices (Holter ECG).

The installation of electrodes should imply prolonged contact with the patient's skin; therefore, special electrically conductive collodion-based adhesives are used as a contact medium. The use of standard gels for outpatient EEG monitoring is not suitable, and the use of conductive pastes is possible only within the daily study.

The time of the study is from 1 day to a week.

After installing the electrodes, they are connected to the device. The operator checks the charge of the power sources of the device, checks the fullness of the information storage, and controls the impedance. After these manipulations, the device is fixed on the patient's body, eliminating tension and breakage of the conductors.

The subject is given a form of a diary of observations drawn up in a free form in which he must enter information about his current condition.

**Important!**

The main task of long-term EEG examinations is to PROVE THE DIRECT RELATIONSHIP of the functional disorders present in the subject with epileptic changes in bioelectrical activity or to prove the absence of this connection!

A successful examination is only one in which a functional disorder was recorded videographically, which forms the basis of the clinical picture of the disease and a clear connection was established between the fact of its occurrence and the registration of pathological paroxysmal activity on the electroencephalogram!!!

If there is no event registration or there is no direct connection between the clinical manifestations of the disease and changes in the electroencephalogram, the results of VideoEEG monitoring are not conclusive!

## 5.6 EEG examination in patients with stroke

Ischemic stroke is a disease that occurs as a result of cerebral infarction and is characterized by the development of persistent focal neurological syndromes of loss of functions, primarily motor.

Therefore, a functional study of the state of the bioelectrical activity of the brain under conditions of motor load is of great interest both in assessing the general condition and in developing rehabilitation measures.

**The purpose of the study** was to evaluate changes in the bioelectrical activity of the brain caused by violations of cerebral hemoperfusion and to identify the reactions of the microcirculatory vascular bed under conditions of physical exertion.

### 5.7 Periodization of ischemic stroke

1. the most acute period—the first 3 days (with regression of symptoms in the first 24 hours, a transient ischemic attack is diagnosed)

2. acute period—up to 21 days

3. early recovery period—up to 6 months

4. late recovery period—up to 2 years

5. period of residual effects—after 2 years

## 6. Mounting 25 active EEG electrodes (as element of “10-10” system)

Volumetric intracerebral processes are characterized by suppression of neuronal activity (especially in the early stages of development). On the EEG, this is reflected in the registration of slow-wave activity, which is poorly localized using the 10-20 system.

To address this issue, in 2017, the International Federation of Clinical Neurophysiology (IFCN) recommended a system of 25 active electrodes in a 10-10 electrode system as the research standard. This system includes 25 active electrodes, against 19 in the standard “10-20” system, which is achieved by introducing three pairs of additional electrodes F9–F10, T9–T10, P9–P10, which allow recording biopotentials from the basal parts of the brain.

### 6.1 Procedure for converting a “10-20” system to a “10-10” system

The procedure for converting the “10-20” system to the “10-10” system includes the introduction of six additional electrodes into the wiring diagram: F9 T9 P9 and F10 T10 P10, one row down (20% of the nasion-inion distance) from the F7 T3 T5 electrodes F8 T4 T6 (**Table 1**).

| Device socket | Electrode |
|---|---|
| X1 | F9 |
| X2 | F10 |
| X3 | T9 |
| X4 | T10 |
| X5 | P9 |
| X6 | P10 |

**Table 1**
*Electrode connections accordingly, the device uses sockets.*

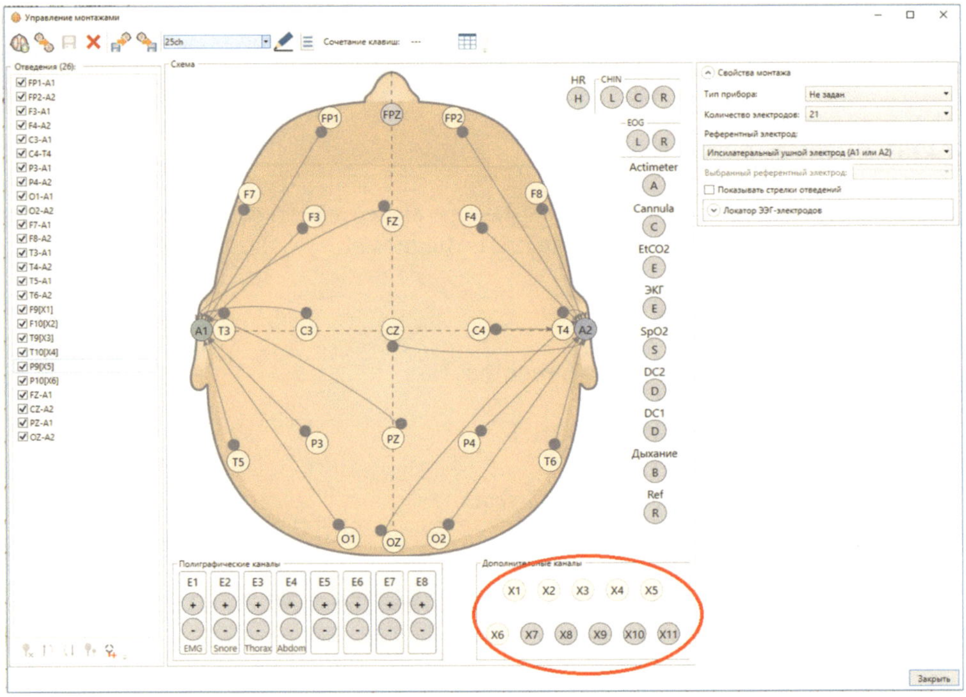


**Figure 1.**
*An example of creating a system 10-10 using additional channels of the device (Program "Neuron-Spectrum" LLC "Neurosoft," Russia, author's observation).*

Instrument socket Electrode X1 F9 X2 F10 X3 T9 X4 T10 X5 P9 X6 P10 For registration, an appropriate new mounting of electrodes is created (**Figure 1**).

## 7. Features of the examination when using a multichannel EEG system

A traditional study with 21 scalp electrodes in a 10-20 system is carried out using simple electrode attachment systems, most often in the form of "caps" of intertwined elastic tubes or cords, and "bridge" electrodes, in which improved skin-electrode contact is achieved using physical solution. This is the so-called classical or "wet" EEG interface. Direct installation of electrodes on the scalp is also possible using needle electrodes or adhesive electrodes attached to the scalp with a paste or collodion gel. This system is used in cases of long recordings and sleep studies. In recent years, the "dry interface" system has been actively introduced, which does not require the use of conductive solutions, pastes, or gels. Each electrode of such a system has a chlorine-silver comb installed directly on the scalp, and the contact error is solved either by a larger electrode surface or by installing a signal microamplifier.

The classical EEG scenario represents a successive change in the recording of background activity and functional tests "on tape" or in one file, which allows the researcher to "scroll the record" to compare the characteristics of the bioelectrical activity of the brain under different conditions and under different external influences. Since the number of electrodes is small, and the distance between them is from 4 to 7 cm, then in such a system there are no strict requirements for determining the spatial location of each electrode.

However, the use of a multichannel system with more than 64 electrodes requires a more careful approach to creating a scalp-electrode system. A small distance between the electrodes of 1–2 cm requires careful use of solutions and gels, since with an overabundance of the latter, a common contact will occur between two adjacent electrodes and, accordingly, they will be "turned off" from the common recording system.

When using a 64-channel system, systems of ring electrodes pumped with an electrically conductive gel are more often used, but when using 128- and 256-channel systems, it is difficult to implement such a solution, since a large number of adjacent electrodes create the problem of forming "conductive bridges" and shorting adjacent electrodes to each other.

The next problem of the multichannel interface is the spatial localization of the electrodes. As mentioned earlier, the use of the 10-20 system and the use of visual-phenomenological analysis allow the researcher to do without this information or use the simplest methods of approximation by the area-electrode type. But the high-density system operates with a much larger number of electrodes located above the same zone, and the researcher uses various methods of analysis that require adequate consideration of differences and input data.

To solve this problem, both methods of a spherical model are currently used with the representation of the head as a sphere of a given radius with a uniform arrangement of electrodes on its surface, as well as more accurate methods of geodetic photogrammetry, which determines the position of the electrode from a series of spatial images with the construction of an individual three-dimensional model, or the method an electronic pointer that allows you to determine the position of the electrode and its connection with the brain structure obtained using the transformation of CT or MRI images (**Figure 2**).

## 8. Problems of visual representation of a multichannel EEG study

When trying to visually and phenomenologically analyze a multichannel EEG recording, it is difficult to identify individual diagnostically significant patterns, since

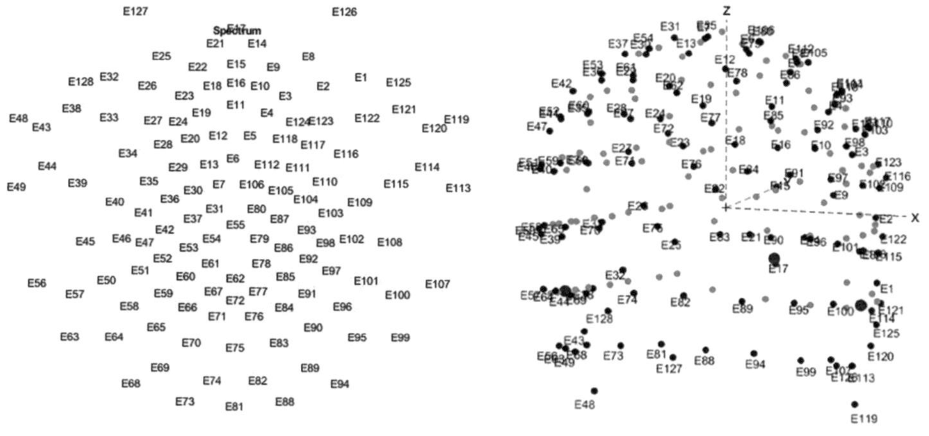


**Figure 2.**
*Spatial localization of 128 electrodes of a multichannel EEG system using a spherical head model (EEGLAB®, author's observation).*

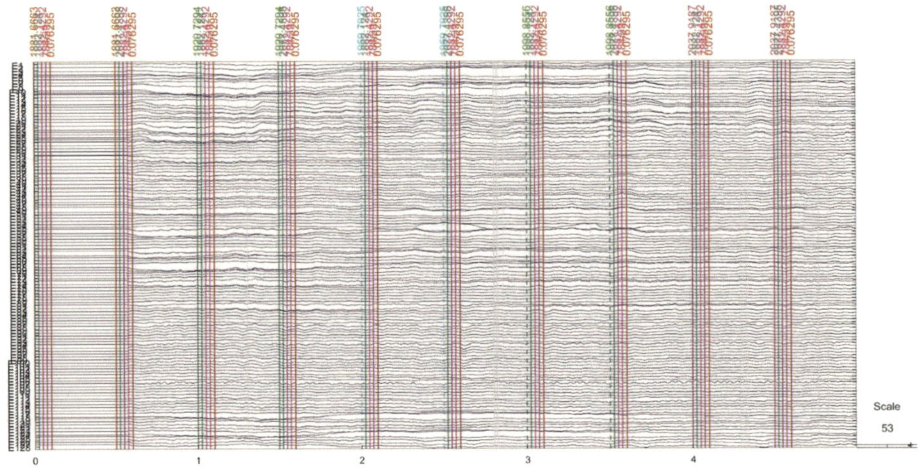


**Figure 3.**
*Visual representation of native recording of 128 channels of EEG recording (EEGLAB®, author's observation).*

a large amount of linear data is located in a limited space, so attempts to identify dynamic changes in bioelectrical activity under these conditions are doomed to failure in advance (**Figure 3**).

It is more rational to use mathematical processing of primary data with the presentation of results in the form of frequency graphs and amplitude-frequency maps (**Figure 4**) [13, 14].

This approach makes it possible to identify functional changes in the bioelectrical activity of the brain by the type of potentials associated with the event, the use of a large number of electrodes that create a dense network allows not only to fix the response to the event, but also to see the reaction of adjacent cortical zones.

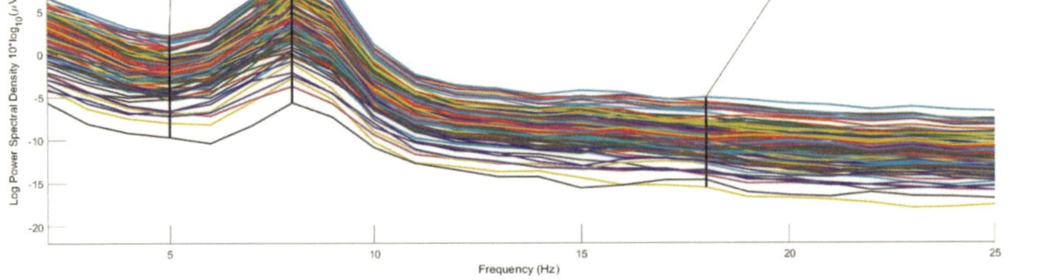


**Figure 4.**
*Mathematical analysis of the native recording, which allows to determine the area of desynchronization of the sensorimotor zone (EEGLAB®, author's observation).*

## 9. The functional study

In the most acute and early recovery period, the patient's condition is still unstable, because the cerebral blood supply system is being restructured, damaged as a result of occlusion of the cerebral arteries and the formation of a compensating collateral blood supply system.

Under these conditions, the determination of changes in the bioelectrical activity of the brain is directly related to disorders of cerebral microcirculation. Since the nerve cell does not have in its structure organelles containing a supply of nutrients, any change in the conditions of its blood supply leads to disturbances in the formation of action potential (AP) and postsynaptic potential (PSP), which is manifested by the appearance of slow-wave activity in the structure of the EEG recording.

To determine the change in the characteristics of bioelectrical activity, we will compare the state of passive relaxed wakefulness and physical activity in the form of rhythmic squeezing—unclenching the hands (**Figure 5**).

In a state of passive relaxed wakefulness, a zone of slow-wave activity of theta—range is recorded in the left frontotemporal leads. A preserved motor area in the right hemisphere of the brain and a shift in the focus of alpha activity to the undamaged hemisphere are determined (**Figures 6** and **7**).

At the beginning of the load, a change in bioelectrical activity is observed, which is characterized by the appearance of a section of slow waves in the frontal regions of the right (intact) hemisphere of the brain, which is a reflection of the formation of a collateral flow along the system of the anterior communicating artery and the steal syndrome of the frontal regions of the healthy hemisphere.

At the third minute of the exercise test in the affected hemisphere, a pronounced increase in the area of slow-wave activity is observed, which characterizes

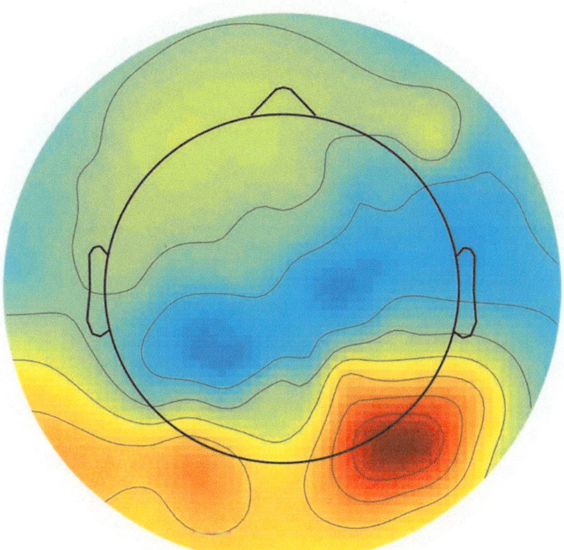

**Figure 5.**
*The state of passive relaxed wakefulness in a patient with ischemic stroke in the basin of the left middle cerebral artery (EEGLAB®, author's observation).*

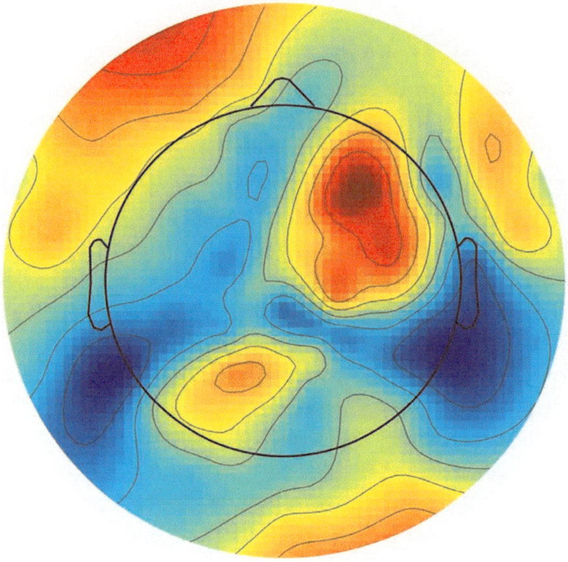

**Figure 6.**
*Formation of areas of low-frequency pathological activity in a patient who started the exercise test (EEGLAB®, author's observation).*

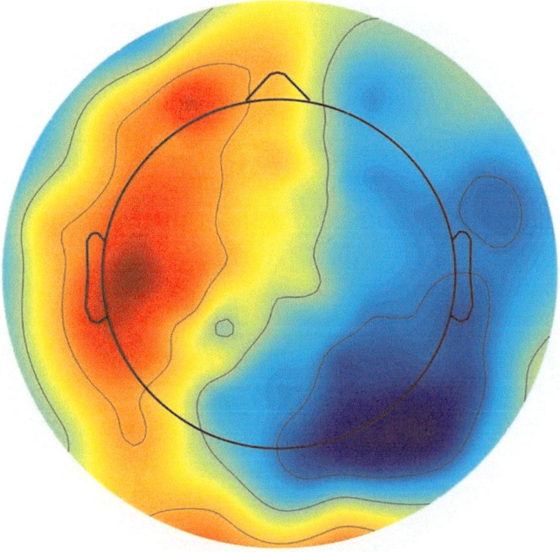

**Figure 7.**
*Continued changes in the characteristics of bioelectrical activity by the end of 3 minutes of functional exercise testing (EEGLAB®, authors observation).*

pronounced microcirculation disorders due to decompensation of the collateral blood supply system. At the same time, the patient does not complain about the deterioration of the general condition.

This observation is important for the development of exercise programs at the early stages of medical rehabilitation, since, as shown above, even slight physical activity can cause decompensation of the emerging collateral blood supply system in such patients.

## 10. Formation of an EEG conclusion

### 10.1 Routine EEG study

Conclusion (Report) is the main result of the study, which characterizes all its importance as a diagnostic method. The report is compiled by the medical specialist who conducted the study and should include the following sections:

Section 1 Guide containing.

- Information of the referring physician (brief description of the patient's condition)
- Patient identification number in the clinic registration system
- Age
- Diagnosis
- Neurological status
- Treatment
- Date of last seizure (in case of examination of a patient with epilepsy)
- Clinical question of the attending physician to be answered by the study

Section 2. Technical

- Information from EEG technician
- Nr. EEG
- Time and date of recording
- Level of consciousness, wakefulness, cooperation with the patient
- Activation procedures used in the study (photostimulation, hyperventilation, mental activation, sensory stimuli, etc.)
- Section 3 Description
- The description of the EEG is carried out using the terminology of the EEG glossary)

- The use of special electrodes during application is noted (basal, nasal, and other additional, conditions for their attachment)
- Recording conditions are indicated—wakefulness / sleep / stupor / coma

3.1. Background activity

- Description of alpha—activity: severity, localization, distribution to the central and frontal leads, amplitude, frequency, frequency modality (monomodal, bimodal, polymodal) severity of amplitude modulations, interhemispheric asymmetry is or is not.
- Description of beta activity, severity, localization, distribution to the posterior leads, amplitude, frequency, interhemispheric asymmetry, whether or not.
- Slow activity Theta and Delta waves
- Severity in leads, type, localization, formation of groups of waves, and pathological rhythms with indication of localization.
- Paroxysmal activity if present
- Appearance of non-epileptiform/epileptiform, bilaterally synchronous, focal, main pathological pattern, its amplitude, frequency, presence/absence of amplitude, and frequency gradients.
- Special EEG patterns (if available)

3.2. Recording under stimulation conditions

- The effect of the activation procedure (opening-closing the eyes)
- Reaction to the test with photostimulation:
    - Rhythm learning yes/no, whether the test provokes the appearance of paroxysmal/epileptiform patterns in the recording. If they are present, a description of their amplitude, frequency, presence/absence of gradients in amplitude and frequency.
- Response to hyperventilation
    - The time of the test is indicated (3, 5, 3+2 min, or the test is terminated at ... a minute).
    - Whether the trial induces paroxysmal/epileptiform patterns in the recording. If they are present, a description of their amplitude, frequency, presence/absence of gradients in amplitude and frequency.

**Important**

- **The normal hyperventilation response implies disorganization and flattening of rhythms for 1 minute of HB, as well as an increase in the index**

**of slow waves in the theta range for 2–3 minutes conducting a sample on the index up to 40% of the epoch.**

- **In children and adolescents, for 2–3 minutes of HB, high-amplitude paroxysmal bioelectrical activity may appear in the form of flashes of bilaterally synchronous waves of the alpha-theta-range, maximally expressed in amplitude in the fronto-central leads (the phenomenon of "respiratory waves" associated with functional immaturity mid-stem structures and their hypersensitivity to hypoxia).**

Section 4. Final

- In this section, the physician makes a judgment by interpreting the data obtained using clinical terminology. The interpretation of the results of the recording is carried out in the context of the diagnosis and the question of the referring physician (clinical significance of the results, prognosis, etc.) using general clinical terms; special EEG terminology should be avoided if possible.

### 10.2 Continued EEG study

Section 1 Guide containing.

- Information of the referring physician (brief description of the patient's condition)
- Patient identification number in the clinic registration system
- Age
- Diagnosis
- Neurological status
- Treatment
- Date of last seizure (in case of examination of a patient with epilepsy)
- Clinical question of the attending physician to be answered by the study
- Section 2. Technical
- Information from EEG technician
- Num. EEG
- Time and date of recording
- Level of consciousness, wakefulness, cooperation with the patient
- Activation procedures used in the study (photostimulation, hyperventilation, mental activation, sensory stimuli, etc.)

Section 3 Description

- The description of the EEG is carried out using the terminology of the EEG glossary)
- The use of special electrodes during application is noted (basal, nasal, and other additional, conditions for their attachment)
- Recording conditions are indicated—wakefulness / sleep / stupor / coma

3.1. Background activity

- Description of alpha—activity: severity, localization, distribution to the central and frontal leads, amplitude, frequency, frequency modality (monomodal, bimodal, polymodal) severity of amplitude modulations, interhemispheric asymmetry is or is not.
- Description of beta activity, severity, localization, distribution to the posterior leads, amplitude, frequency, interhemispheric asymmetry, whether or not.
- Slow activity Theta and Delta waves
- Severity in leads, type, localization, formation of groups of waves and pathological rhythms with indication of localization.
- Paroxysmal activity if present
- Appearance non-epileptiform/epileptiform, bilaterally synchronous, focal, main pathological pattern, its amplitude, frequency, presence/absence of amplitude, and frequency gradients.
- Special EEG patterns (if available)
- 3.2. Recording under stimulation conditions

**Important!**
**We note the number of stimulation tests in the study and the patient's condition during their execution**

3.2. The effect of the activation procedure (opening-closing the eyes)

- Reaction to the test with photostimulation:
    - Rhythm learning yes/no, whether the test provokes the appearance of paroxysmal/epileptiform patterns in the recording. If they are present, a description of their amplitude, frequency, presence/absence of gradients in amplitude and frequency.
- Response to hyperventilation
    - The time of the test is indicated (3, 5, 3+2 min, or the test is terminated at ... a minute).

- Whether the trial induces paroxysmal/epileptiform patterns in the recording. If they are present, a description of their amplitude, frequency, presence/absence of gradients in amplitude and frequency.

**Important**

- **The normal hyperventilation response implies disorganization and flattening of rhythms for 1 minute of HB, as well as an increase in the index of slow waves in the theta range for 2–3 minutes conducting a sample on the index up to 40% of the epoch.**
- **In children and adolescents, for 2–3 minutes of HB, high-amplitude paroxysmal bioelectrical activity may appear in the form of flashes of bilaterally synchronous waves of the alpha-theta-range, maximally expressed in amplitude in the fronto-central leads (the phenomenon of "respiratory waves" associated with functional immaturity mid-stem structures and their hypersensitivity to hypoxia).**

**Important**

**If an epileptic seizure develops or the patient refuses to continue the procedure, stop the study**

**Section 4. Final**

**In this section, the physician makes a judgment by interpreting the data obtained using clinical terminology. The interpretation of the results of the recording is carried out in the context of the diagnosis and the question of the referring physician (clinical significance of the results, prognosis, etc.) using general clinical terms; special EEG terminology should be avoided if possible.**

### 10.3 Video EEG monitoring

Section 1 Guide containing.

- Information of the referring physician (brief description of the patient's condition)
- Patient identification number in the clinic registration system
- Age
- Diagnosis
- Neurological status
- Treatment
- Date of last seizure (in case of examination of a patient with epilepsy)
- Clinical question of the attending physician to be answered by the study

Section 2. Technical

- Information from EEG technician
- Num. EEG
- Time and date of recording
- Level of consciousness, wakefulness, cooperation with the patient
- Time of arrival of the patient at the clinic
- Time of arrival of the patient in the ward
- Bed time
- Light off time
- Sleep time
- Total sleep time
- Number of awakenings
- Light on time
- Wake up time
- Study termination time
- Time of patient leaving the clinic

Section 3 Description

- The description of the EEG is carried out using the terminology of the EEG glossary)
- The use of special electrodes during application is noted (basal, nasal, and other additional, conditions for their attachment)
- Recording conditions are specified
    - Awake
    - Sandman
    - NREM 1
    - NREM sleep phase 2
- upon reaching

- Stage 3 slow-wave sleep
- 4th phase of non-REM sleep
- 5 REM sleep

3.1. Waking with open eyes

- The presence of oculograms and muscle artifacts is noted

3.2. Waking with closed eyes

- Description of alpha activity: severity, localization, distribution to the central and frontal leads, amplitude, frequency, frequency modality (monomodal, bimodal, polymodal) severity of amplitude modulations, interhemispheric asymmetry is or is not.
- Description of beta activity, severity, localization, distribution to the posterior leads, amplitude, frequency, interhemispheric asymmetry, whether or not.
- Slow activity Theta and Delta waves
- Severity in leads, type, localization, formation of groups of waves and pathological rhythms with indication of localization.
- Paroxysmal activity if present
- Appearance non-epileptiform/epileptiform, bilaterally synchronous, focal, main pathological pattern, its amplitude, frequency, presence/absence of amplitude and frequency gradients.
- Special EEG patterns (if available)

3.3. Sandman

- Flattening of rhythms is noted. The appearance of lambda waves in the occipital leads, oculographic artifact and myographic artifacts from shudders can be recorded.
- The period of drowsiness can move into a state of passive relaxed wakefulness with eyes closed and can move into phase 1 of non-REM sleep.

3.4. 1 slow-wave sleep (non-REM I)

- The flattening of rhythmic activity, characteristic of the state of drowsiness, persists. Lambda waves are absent in the frontal leads, a spindle-shaped sigma appears—a rhythm with a frequency of 16–22 Hz. Amplitude up to 30 microvolts.

- Phase 1 slow-wave sleep can move into a state of passive relaxed wakefulness with eyes closed and can move into phase 2 slow-wave sleep.

3.4. NREM 2 (non-REM II)

- The flattening of rhythmic activity is preserved. Lambda waves are absent in the frontal leads, a spindle-shaped sigma appears—a rhythm with a frequency of 16–22 Hz.
- In the central-parietal leads, paroxysmal activity is recorded in the form of bilateral-synchronous polyphasic complexes with an amplitude of up to 100 microvolts (Vertex-potentials).
- There is an increase in the index of theta range waves up to 30% in the recording epoch, the appearance of groups of theta waves.
- 2nd phase of non-REM sleep can go into a state of passive relaxed wakefulness with eyes closed and can go into phase 3 of slow-wave sleep.

3.5. NREM 3 (non-REM III)

- There is an increase in the index of theta waves in the range of more than 30% in the recording epoch, the appearance of groups of theta waves and unstable rhythms. Bilaterally synchronous delta waves of high amplitude up to 40% are recorded in the recording epoch.
- Sigma—the rhythm is not expressed, the vertex potentials are preserved, but the index is less than in the second phase of non-REM sleep.
- NREM phase 3 can transition into NREM sleep 1 or 2.
- 3.6. 4 phase slow sleep (non-REM IV)
- There is an increase in the delta wave index of more than 60% in the epoch. Delta activity is a bilaterally synchronous rhythm
- Sigma—the rhythm is not expressed, the vertex potentials are not expressed.
- NREM 4 can progress to NREM 3 or 2.

### 3.7. REM sleep phase (REM V)

- Most often achieved in the second half of the night. It is characterized by flattening of background activity to the level of beta with the appearance of multiple oculographic artifacts of different directions. Vertex potentials and sigma rhythm are present but less pronounced than in the second phase of non-REM sleep

**Important!**

- **In each of the phases,**

- **The type of brain activity characteristic of this phase.**
- **Artifacts**
- **Nonspecific and specific sleep phenomena**
- **Paroxysmal and epileptiform changes, if any (indicating localization, amplitude and frequency)**

### 10.4 Ambulatory monitoring

Section 1 Guide containing.

- Information of the referring physician (brief description of the patient's condition)
- Patient identification number in the clinic registration system
- Age
- Diagnosis
- Neurological status
- Treatment
- Date of last seizure (in case of examination of a patient with epilepsy)
- Clinical question of the attending physician to be answered by the study

Section 2. Technical

- Information from EEG technician
- Num. EEG
- Time and date of recording
- Level of consciousness, wakefulness, cooperation with the patient
- Time of arrival of the patient at the clinic
- Machine start time
- Total recording time (days)
- Time of removal of the research apparatus
- Time of patient leaving the clinic

Section 3 Description

- The description of the EEG is carried out using the terminology of the EEG glossary)
- The use of special electrodes during application is noted (basal, nasal, and other additional, conditions for their attachment)
- Recording conditions are indicated in accordance with the diary entries of the subject
- Assess the association of registered changes with disturbances in daily activities
- When fixing epileptic seizures, their impact on the quality of life of the subject is assessed

**Important!**
**With long-term outpatient monitoring, it is necessary to organize control over the state of electrode connection!**

## 11. Conclusion

The study of the functional activity of the brain remains the most important problem in clinical neurophysiology. But for its solution, it requires the combined efforts of specialists from different areas of neuroscience and is unthinkable without the improvement of methods that make it possible to fix, localize, and understand the processes occurring in the nervous tissue.

The EEG method developed at the beginning of the twentieth century still retains its relevance in the clinic of neurological diseases. The main and most demanded advantage of the EEG method is the possibility of direct study of the bioelectrical activity of brain structures, which makes it possible to study processes with rapid dynamics occurring in brain structures.

Nevertheless, methodological approaches to the analysis of electroencephalograms need a thorough revision and the formation of a unified methodological approach to the implementation of research, especially with the active introduction of multichannel systems combined with computer signal processing into clinical practice, which in the future can change many ideas about the pathogenesis of various neurological diseases and suggest the most rational approaches to their therapy and rehabilitation.

## Author details

Sergey Alexander Gulyaev
National Research Nuclear University (MEPHI) Engineering Physics Institute of Biomedicine, Moscow, Russia

*Address all correspondence to: sergruss@yandex.ru

## References

[1] Kulaichev AP. Computer electrophysiology and functional diagnostics. Ed. 4th, revised. and additional - M.: INFRA-M. 2007. pp. 178-230. ISBN 978-5-16-014671-3 (RUS)

[2] Penfield U, Roberts L. Speech and brain mechanisms L. Medicine. 1964; **1964**:264

[3] Roterman-Konieczna I. Simulations in Medicine: Computer-aided diagnostics and therapy. Berlin, Boston: De Gruyter; 2020

[4] Ryynänen OR, Hyttinen JA, Malmivuo JA. Effect of measurement noise and electrode density on the spatial resolution of cortical potential distribution with different resistivity values for the skull. IEEE Transaction on Biomedical Engineering. 2006;**53**(9): 1851-1858

[5] Lantz G, Grave de Peralta R, Spinelli L, Seeck M, Michel CM. Epileptic source localization with high density EEG: How many electrodes are needed? Clinical Neurophysiology. 2003; **114**(1):63-69

[6] Wójcik GM. 3 Selected methods of quantitative analysis in electroencephalography. In: Roterman-Konieczna I, editor. Simulations in Medicine: Computer-aided diagnostics and therapy. Berlin, Boston: De Gruyter; 2020. pp. 35-54

[7] Pascual-Marqui RD, Esslen M, Kochi K, Lehmann D. Functional imaging with low-resolution brain electromagnetic tomography (LORETA): A review. Methods in Experimental Clinical Pharmacology. 2002; **24**(Suppl. C):91-95

[8] Seeck M, Koessler L, Bast T, Leijten F, Michel C, Baumgartner C, et al. The standardized EEG electrode array of the IFCN. Clinical Neurophysiology. 2017; **128**(10):2070-2077

[9] Rossini PM, Di Iorio R, Bentivoglio M, Bertini G, Ferreri F, Gerloff C, et al. Methods for analysis of brain connectivity: An IFCN-sponsored review. Clinical Neurophysiology. 2019; **130**(10):1833-1858

[10] Stergiadis C, Kostaridou VD, Veloudis S, Kazis D, Klados MA. A personalized user authentication system based on EEG signals. Sensors (Basel). 2022;**22**(18):6929

[11] Romeo Z, Mantini D, Durgoni E, Passarini L, Meneghello F, Zorzi M. Electrophysiological signatures of resting state networks predict cognitive deficits in stroke. Cortex. 2021;**138**:59-71

[12] Manganotti P, Furlanis G, Ajčević M, Polverino P, Caruso P, Ridolfi M, et al. CT perfusion and EEG patterns in patients with acute isolated aphasia in seizure-related stroke mimics. Seizure. 2019;**71**:110-115

[13] Delorme A, Sejnowski T, Makeig S. Enhanced detection of artifacts in EEG data using higher-order statistics and independent component analysis. NeuroImage. 2007;**34**:4

[14] Tadel F, Baillet S, Mosher JC, Pantazis D, Leahy RM. Brainstorm: A user-friendly application for MEG/EEG analysis. Computer in Intellectual Neuroscience. 2011;**2011**:879716

Chapter 2

# Neuroimaging for Epilepsy Diagnosis and Management

*Lau Sau Ning Sarah, Cheng King Fai Kevin and Grace Ho*

## Abstract

This chapter will cover the neuroimaging techniques and their application to the diagnostic work up and management of adults and children with new onset or chronic epilepsy. We will focus on the specific indications and requirements of different imaging techniques for the diagnosis and pre-surgical work up of pharmacoresistant focal epilepsies. We will discuss the sensitivity, specificity and prognostic value of imaging features, benign variants and artefacts, and the possible diagnostic significance of non-epileptogenic lesions. This chapter is intended to be relevant for day-to-day practice in average clinical circumstances, with emphasis on MRI and most commonly used functional neuroimaging techniques.

**Keywords:** MRI, epilepsy, temporal, extratemporal, SPECT, PET

## 1. Introduction

The advent of neuroimaging has provided powerful tools for the identification of epileptogenic lesions preoperatively. This has increased the number of surgical candidates and improved postsurgical outcomes [1–3]. The approach of presurgical evaluation in patients with potential epileptogenic lesions has also radically changed, absolving the need for invasive neurophysiologic techniques.

Magnetic resonance imaging is currently the best available tool for identification of epileptogenic lesions, newer scanning techniques such as 3T magnets, functional MRI (fMRI), and diffusion tensor imaging (DTI) are giving clinicians more insight into the presumptive pathology. More importantly these techniques allow precise 3D anatomic localization of the lesion and its relationship to adjacent structures and network connectivity (brain connectome). Novel imaging results are giving us more information about cortical function and/or dysfunction in patients with epilepsy in order to predict postoperative deficits and odds of seizure freedom. This has given a lot of hope to patients previously diagnosed with refractory epilepsy with no identifiable culprit.

## 2. MRI

3T MRI scanners are now widely available and replacing 1.5T scanners for epilepsy protocol imaging. Increase in the magnetic field strength in 3T MRI improves the signal-to-noise ratio and contrast-to-noise ratio, thereby improving the detection of elusive lesions such as malformations of cortical development (MCD) [4–7]. Challenges of ultra-high-field imaging include far greater radiofrequency signal inhomogeneities, higher energy deposition in tissue, and more pronounced imaging artifacts at soft tissue–air and soft tissue–bone interfaces. 3T MRI also has increased device incompatibility [4, 8, 9] compared to older machines.

Most MRI studies for evaluation of epilepsy would first include a sagittal T1-weighted spin-echo acquisition in order to position the slices of the subsequent pulse sequences. Two kinds of protocols were commonly used in epilepsy imaging in the past, the temporal lobe protocol and extratemporal protocol. However, these protocols would often neglect substantial parts of the non-targeted area of the brain. Some centres now advocate a more comprehensive protocol [10, 11]. Supplementary imaging sequences include T2* gradient echo, DWI, sagittal 3D TSE T2/FLAIR, contrast imaging and post-processing techniques such as voxel based morphometry. FLAIR has a specific advantage over T2 for lesions in periventricular, hippocampal and subpial cortex locations due to proximity to the brain-CSF interface. Other lesions readily identified by FLAIR include subtle hyperintensities blurring the gray-white junction of MCD, subcortical foci of gliotic hyperintensity in areas of encephalomalacia, and the extent of infiltration of low-grade neoplasms. Limitations of FLAIR include CSF pulsation induced motion artifacts causing blurring of the medial temporal regions and contrast suppression obscuring visualization of small foci of heterotopic gray matter. Also of note is that contrast on fast FLAIR seems to be most limiting in patients with immature white matter i.e. young children (<2 years). Conventional spin density images tend to be more helpful in this age group.

Signal characteristics of immature myelin in infants and young children can pose significant challenges in interpretation of studies obtained in infancy. Lesions such as MCDs and cortical tubers have varying signal characteristics depending on the developmental stage of the myelin of the lesions and the surrounding brain. In infants, the dysplastic cortex and adjacent subcortical regions may appear hypointense on T2-weighted images and hyperintense on T1 sequences, contrary to the reverse pattern seen in older children and adults [12–14]. In some patients these lesions tend to become less obvious or rarely "vanish" on follow-up imaging [15] thus reviewing only the most recent images may fail to detect the lesions. Conversely, a "new lesion" of MCD may be detected on follow-up imaging due to the poor background contrast of the bright immature myelin on the T2 images [16]. Follow-up MRI during 2nd year of life or later may unmask areas of MCD with decreased or absent subcortical myelin. Cortical tubers of tuberous sclerosis may be more evident on follow-up imaging. Apart from changes in myelination, increased growth of tubers and dystrophic calcification may contribute to their better visibility on follow-up imaging. Serial MRIs are helpful in other epileptic disorders such as Rasmussen encephalitis and Sturge-Weber syndrome to demonstrate progressive regional or hemispheric cortical atrophy.

### 2.1 Susceptibility weight imaging (SWI)

SWI techniques exploit differences in magnetic susceptibility of tissue components such as deoxygenated blood, iron, and calcium to provide additional information in epileptogenic lesions containing blood products. This can be useful for cavernomas, certain posttraumatic epilepsies, and Sturge-Weber syndrome. SWI is superior to T2* Gradient Echo (GRE) in detection of remote hemorrhages. Cortical gyral abnormalities in Sturge-Weber syndrome can represent venous stasis-related hypoxia, and their SWI findings seem to correspond to the hypometabolic areas detected on FDG-PET. Thus, SWI has the potential to show functional information in addition to anatomical details in Sturge-Weber syndrome [17, 18].

### 2.2 Diffusion weighted imaging (DWI)

One of the more commonly encountered techniques in MRI is DWI. DWI was initially introduced in clinical practice for the early detection of stroke as it is very sensitive to areas affected by ischemia [19]. Animal studies on status epilepticus have highlighted initial restricted diffusion due to cytotoxic edema and, after several days, to normalization or facilitated diffusion [20–23]. Diffusion imaging may, therefore, provide an opportunity to directly image the areas involved in seizure generation and possibly spread. Overall, the correlation between the presumed epileptogenic zone and the diffusion changes is quite variable. In focal epilepsies, peri-ictal isolated low ADC values without overt hyperintensity on DWI have been reported. Peri-ictal cytotoxic edema with foci of hyperintensity on DWI with decreased ADC values have also been reported [24–26]. Correlations seem closer in patients with longer seizures (or status) and short duration between seizure end and scan [24, 27]. In contrast, interictal neuronal loss and increased extracellular space have been reflected in increased ADC values. Other disorders related to epilepsy that may show DWI abnormalities include cortical and subcortical abnormalities in status epilepticus, antiseizure medications and transient lesions of splenium of corpus callosum related to seizures [28–30]. A significant increase in ADC has been reported in epileptogenic tubers in patients with tuberous sclerosis.

### 2.3 Diffusion tensor imaging (DTI) and tractography

Diffusion tensor imaging (DTI) allows measurement of water diffusion in order to provide information on microstructural changes and connections between different regions of the brain. Animal models have revealed myelin as the main barrier to water diffusion [31–34]. This allows interrogation of white matter architecture and morphological reconstruction of major tracts in vivo. This method is still quite crude, however, and cannot resolve distinct fibers that cross within a voxel. White matter tractography is generally done in two different ways, either with a method known as "deterministic" tractography or with a "probabilistic" method. Using deterministic methods, points are placed, and the tract grows in both directions along the dominant diffusion direction. The probabilistic method probe fiber orientation distributions at each voxel and is computationally more intensive but can more reliably reconstruct crossing fibers.

The objective of epilepsy surgery in pharmacoresistant focal epilepsies is complete resection or at least disconnection of the epileptogenic zone while preserving eloquent cortex [2, 35]. Exploring white matter changes in epilepsy can help us to understand epileptogenicity, they may also be a surrogate marker for cognitive difficulties and can inform clinicians about risks of epilepsy surgery procedures. Once successfully implemented into neuronavigation systems this information may also be used intraoperatively to tailor resections [36]. Extratemporal surgeries will also benefit from visualizing crucial connections and tracts such as the pyramidal tract. Implementation of DTI-based tractography has already been shown to benefit patients undergoing brain tumor surgeries and resections of vascular malformations [36–40] and will certainly be increasingly used in epilepsy surgery.

### 2.4 fMRI

The simultaneous recording of electroencephalogram (EEG) and functional MRI (fMRI) was first demonstrated in patients with epilepsy in the early 1990s and has since become an important research tool in epilepsy and beyond [41]. EEG-fMRI has been primarily used as a localization technique. In addition it can be combined with other more advanced modeling methodologies to study the networks connectivity. Together, both technologies may allow for novel insights in understanding the ictal-onset zone, irritative zone, and functional deficit zone (the connectome).

### 2.5 Ultra-high-field 7T MRI

The first 7T MRI scanner was FDA approved for clinical diagnostic use in October 2017. 7T MRI is currently available for use in few centers. Improved image resolution and contrast at 7T, especially with the MP2RAGE sequence [42] opens new possibilities for visualization of internal details of hippocampal subfields [43]. Although the clinical yield of 7T visual analysis on 3T-negative cases was still unclear in TLE, studies utilizing quantitative approaches have suggested promising results [44, 45]. 7T MRI can lead to better detection of FCD in ETLE, even in some cases with negative 3T MRI [46–52]. The availability of higher magnetic field strength does not preclude the combined use of advanced image postprocessing to optimize diagnostic yields.

### 2.6 MRI postprocessing techniques

Several commercial packages enable the quantification of MRI structural features and are currently used in routine clinical practice. FDA-approved software packages include NeuroQuant (Cortechs Labs, San Diego, CA), BrainReader (BrainReader, Denmark), and icobrain (icometrix, Leuven, Belgium). These softwares typically generate a report that details the volume and percentile of each parcellated cortical regions, with comparison to normative databases. In epilepsy, NeuroQuant has been shown to lateralize hippocampal atrophy in TLE patients with accuracy rates that could exceed those achieved with visual inspection of clinical MR imaging studies [53].

Incorporating postprocessing techniques into routine care requires the use of high-quality MRI acquisition with 3D volumetric sequences for optimal results. It also requires specialized expertise in computational anatomy and seamless communication within the multidisciplinary epilepsy team. These techniques can provide unapparelled power in the ability to detect significant epileptogenic brain lesions in surgical candidates. Discovering a previously undetected lesion can drastically change the presurgical planning and surgical outcome. In fact, the lack of a visible lesion has consistently been shown to predict surgical failure [54, 55], and MRI-positive surgical candidates are two times more likely to become seizure free after epilepsy surgery than MRI-negative patients [56].

MCD is generally regarded as the most common epileptogenic substrate that can evade detection. Sometimes the only MRI finding of MCD can just be subtle blurring at the gray–white junction without hyperintensity on T2 or FLAIR. Novel quantitative image analyses can increase the yield of detecting relevant structural lesions in a sensitive, replicable, and reader-independent fashion, significantly complementing conventional visual analysis. Image reconstruction by manual means in a curvilinear plane—a plane parallel to the cortical surface and perpendicular in relation to the gyri—can show progressively deeper surfaces of the brain. This will result in a more uniform distribution of gray matter on both hemispheres assisting in comparison of homologous regions of the cortex [57–59]. In addition to improving the detection of subtle MCDs, such surface reconstructions can also more precisely assess the location of subdural grids and depth electrodes and aid in presurgical planning.

### 2.7 Voxel-based morphometry (VBM)

VBM is one of the most popular and most useful postprocessing algorithms to date. Large-population control averages are used as common reference [60], however, references for adults should not be used to study paediatric cohorts. This fully automated technique extracts gray matter and white matter maps from individuals to make statistical comparisons with respect to a normal database [61]. VBM is able to accentuate abnormalities in the gray-white junction [62], minimizing "false-positive" studies. When there is an a priori hypothesis based on clinical and EEG data to confine the analysis to a certain brain region, VBM can be used to aim for maximal specificity. Whereas when EEG or other functional imaging data do not point to a region of interest, it is essential to opt for maximal sensitivity.

VBM consistently reported gray matter abnormalities extending beyond the visible culprit, sometimes distant from the epileptogenic area [63–66]. These changes could be due to occult dysplastic regions undetectable by visual analysis or represent an abnormal gyration [63]. These clusters may indicate dysplastic abnormalities much more widespread across the hemispheres than the changes visible on the MRI and may explain, at least in part, why in some cases complete resection of MRI lesion does not always lead to seizure freedom. It is also conceivable that these changes may potentially become active at a later stage and cause seizure recurrence after surgery [67].

### 2.8 MRI volumetry

In temporal lobe epilepsy (TLE), the epileptogenic network causes variable degrees of neuronal loss and astrogliosis across hippocampal subfields, the amygdala, and the entorhinal cortex, namely mesial temporal sclerosis (MTS) [68]. In many patients, MTS can be visualized on MRI as noticeable hippocampal atrophy, increased T2-weighted signal, and loss of internal architecture. However, the visual identification of morphologic and signal characteristics of the hippocampus is highly subjective and depends heavily on the experience of the reader. Manual MRI volumetry is a commonly used quantitative technique to assess mesial temporal lobe atrophy, as it has been demonstrated to be more sensitive than visual evaluation [69]. Volumetry of the entorhinal cortex, amygdala, and temporopolar region as well as the thalamus may also assist in lateralization of the seizure focus [70]. Specifically, in patients with a normal-appearing hippocampal structure by visual inspection, volumetry of the entorhinal cortex atrophy can provide accurate lateralization of the seizure focus in 25% of cases [71]. Quantification of mesial temporal structures is strongly recommended in order to detect subtle atrophy or abnormal signal increases ipsilateral to the seizure focus and to assess objectively the integrity of the contralateral structures in preparation for epilepsy surgery. Indeed, bilateral mesial temporal lobe atrophy raises concern of markedly reduced chance of seizure freedom after surgery, and an increased risk of memory impairment.

Volumetry studies have consistently revealed gray matter reduction extending beyond the atrophic hippocampus to the adjacent parahippocampal, frontal and anterior temporal regions, suggesting a disruption of frontolimbic pathways. These widespread abnormalities have been associated with seizure frequency [72], epilepsy duration [73, 74], and cognitive dysfunction [75–78]. Patients with persistent seizures after removal of the hippocampus may also have a more widespread neocortical grey matter volume loss [79, 80].

## 2.9 Sulcal morphometry

Sulcal and gyral abnormalities in ETLE patients are characterized by a spectrum of changes [81–83]. In some instances these sulcal morphologic signs may be the only marker for cortical dysgenesis. It was reported that 85% of small FCD lesions that elude visual inspection are found at the bottom of an abnormally deep sulcus [84]. Such preferential location can be explained by local weakness within the developing cortical mantle, co-occurrence of incomplete maturation, decreased neuronal density, and disrupted connectivity in areas surrounding the FCD [69, 85]. Automated extraction, identification, and statistical analysis of cortical sulci was tested in a small series and small FCDs not detected on routine MRI was found on histopathology, particularly in the depth of the posterosuperior and intermediate frontal sulci [86].

### *2.9.1 Shape analysis*

Visualization of hippocampal shape may extend evaluation to details not evident by measurements of hippocampal volume. This technique showed significant inward deviation in the Sommer sector of the sclerotic hippocampi. The analysis of curvature in the hippocampus also revealed medial bending of the posterior hippocampus in patients with TLE, compared with a superomedial shift of the hippocampal body observed in patients with MCD [87].

An extension of shape analysis to adjacent convexities often shows a pathologic relationship. For example, hippocampal malrotation in TLE is associated with increased complexity of the temporolimbic cortices, encompassing parahippocampal, temporopolar, insular, and fronto-opercular regions. This implies that neurodevelopmental factors may play a role in the epileptogenic process [88].

### *2.9.2 Cortical thickness*

Progressive neocortical thinning in the frontal lobes had been found in patients with ongoing seizures than in patients with controlled seizures [89]. This was subsequently echoed in a meta-analysis that showed more marked atrophy in the ipsilateral hippocampus, with moderate effect sizes, in patients with longer epilepsy duration and more frequent seizures [90].

### *2.9.3 Automatic segmentation*

Increasingly sophisticated automatic segmentation algorithms are developed for the assessment of mesial temporal lobe structures. While the majority of them generally demonstrate an excellent performance in healthy subjects, accuracy in patients drops significantly due to the atypical shape, positioning, and size of the hippocampus secondary to incomplete unfolding (or malrotation which occurs in about 40% of TLE patients) [88, 91, 92]. Automated hippocampal segmentation algorithm which integrates deformable parametric surfaces and multiple templates in a unified framework have been developed [93]. This provides flexibility to model disease-related shape deformations and atrophy and is important in maintaining a high-level performance regardless of the presence of abnormal morphology [94, 95].

#### *2.9.4 T2 relaxation times*

The sensitivity of VBM can be increased by directly mapping T2 relaxation times. In the vast majority of TLE patients with hippocampal atrophy, T2 relaxation times within the hippocampal gray matter ipsilateral to the focus increased by at least 10ms when compared to controls [96–98]. This may allow mapping of lateralizing information in patients with no evidence of atrophy on MRI [99].

#### *2.9.5 Multicontrast frameworks*

The sensitivity to detect lesions undetectable by conventional MRI has been shown to increase proportionally to the number of techniques employed, suggesting that each contrast interrogates specific aspects of tissue structure. The combined sensitivity of various contrasts can be assessed by multivariate framework [69]. This can be used in subtyping of FCD. This method showed that FCD type IIB was characterized by abnormal morphology, intensity, diffusivity, and function across all surfaces, while type IIA lesions presented only with increased FLAIR signal and reduced diffusion anisotropy close to the gray-white interface. This multimodal MRI profiling method shows that normal-appearing cortex surrounding the lesion presents with alterations resembling those found at the lesion center [100]. This may help inform proper estimation of lesion extent.

#### *2.9.6 Multimodal framework*

The advent of MRI has tremendously advanced the field of epilepsy surgery. Various MRI techniques providing information on function and connections of different areas of the brain have helped with surgical planning immensely. However, the clinical utility of these techniques in large patient population has not been studied. To this date, a significant number of patients with refractory partial epilepsy still do not have an identifiable lesion on MRI. In such cases results of structural MRI postprocessing need to be confirmed with modalities that can characterize the pathophysiologic features of suspicious imaging findings. Invasive intracranial monitoring is often required, despite which the outcome remains poor. In the context of presurgical evaluation, localization data acquired from seizure semiology, magnetic source imaging (MSI), EEG, MEG, PET and SPECT may help pinpoint the area of interest. Studies have shown combined features from MRI and PET outperformed MRI postprocessing by itself, PET postprocessing by itself, and multimodal visual analysis [101, 102]. Development of newer MR techniques in the future may also have the potential to improve the understanding of the cytoarchitectural and molecular abnormalities of the brain with a greater impact in the field of epilepsy. Understanding postprocessing-positive structural changes outside the assumed epileptogenic zone will require further correlative studies with electrophysiology, pathology, and long-term surgical follow-up.

## 3. Nuclear imaging (PET, SPECT)

Positron emission tomography (PET) and single photon emission computed tomography (SPECT) utilizes radiotracers, and are performed primarily to identify or confirm the ictal focus in preparation for surgery. PET and SPECT help to investigate the pathophysiology of partial and generalized seizure disorders. Occasionally, PET is performed to identify eloquent cortical regions to be spared during epilepsy surgery.

Radiotracer studies using PET or SPECT allow for in vivo assessment of physiologic function of the brain. Such studies include glucose consumption ([18F]fluoro-2-deoxyglucose; [18F]FDG), cerebral blood flow ([15O]water), neurotransmitter synthesis (dopamine and serotonin), receptor ligand binding (agonists or antagonists to benzodiazepine, opiate, serotonin, and N-methyl-d-aspartate [NMDA] receptors), transporter proteins, and microglia. PET has a practical resolution of 2–3 mm, which is superior to that of SPECT, and can be quantitated. Compound half-lives help decide the use and application of PET ligands: 18F-tagged compounds have a 110-minute half-life, 11C a 20-minute half-life, and 15O a 2-minute half-life. The long half-life of [18F]FDG makes it not a good candidate for assessing short-lived physiologic phenomena such as ictal states, whereas the very short half-life of [15O]water allows it to capture the brief activity of cognitive processes. Given the relatively short half-life of PET ligands, data acquisition must occur shortly or immediately after injection.

### 3.1 PET

The most clinical experience for evaluating patients with partial epilepsy is with [18F]FDG-PET. Studies have demonstrated interictal regional decreases in glucose consumption ipsilateral to the seizure focus that is most pronounced in the temporal lobe [103–105]. This figure is close to 90% on recent generation scanners [106–109]. The area of decreased glucose utilization is often more extensive than the epileptogenic zone, may extend into adjacent inferior frontal or parietal lobe neocortex [105, 110] and occasionally into ipsilateral thalamus [111] and contralateral cerebellum [105].

The reason for regional hypometabolism is incompletely understood. Cell loss resulting in synaptic loss and altered remote projections, or hippocampal atrophy in mesial temporal sclerosis, may account for a portion of regional hypometabolism in TLE [112–114]. Hypometabolism does not correlate with lifetime generalized tonic-clonic (GTC) seizures or complex partial seizure (CPS) frequency [115]. Dysplastic tissue with aberrant synaptic connectivity can have either decreased or normal glucose consumption [116]. In focal cortical dysplasia, mitochondrial complex IV function may be decreased in areas of hypometabolism [117]. The abnormalities in some circumstances appear to be functional, as some patients have profound decreases in glucose uptake and no discernible pathology. In patients with mesial temporal sclerosis, the predominant regions that may manifest decreased glucose consumption are the lateral neocortex and, to a lesser extent, the frontal cortex. This may reflect the distant projection of functional loss in mesial structures. Frontal hypometabolism and contralateral hypometabolism appears to be reversible with successful temporal lobectomy [118]. Patterns of hypometabolism may reflect seizure characteristics and seizure propagation. Nevertheless, there is sufficient variability that individual predictions of seizure focus within the temporal lobe cannot be made based on [18F]FDG-PET alone [119], whereas a combination of MRI and PET findings predicted outcome—those with persistent abnormalities fared less well [120].

Metabolic abnormalities are less common in patients with recent-onset, nonrefractory, or well-controlled partial epilepsy [121]. Regional hypometabolism was also found to be changed in relation to seizure frequency in children with worsening seizures [122]. Similar to adults, 70% of children with chronic partial epilepsy (duration 10 years) have focal metabolic abnormalities. There is evidence that adult patients with a greater duration of epilepsy are more likely to have focal [18F]FDG-PET abnormalities [105, 123, 124]. Partial seizures of greater duration are also associated with a greater dissociation between metabolism and blood flow. These [18F]FDG and cerebral blood flow studies, along with cross-sectional studies using volumetric MRI, may be taken as evidence that TLE in some patients is associated with chronic and continued neuronal injury [106, 125].

Although glucose consumption in temporal cortex is decreased, perfusion is often maintained, especially in lateral neocortex [106, 123]. Interictal studies of cerebral blood flow using [15O]water find a decrease in perfusion in only 50% of patients [106]. These data suggest that vascular tone may be impaired in TLE and that there is dissociation between metabolism and perfusion, rendering interictal blood flow studies unreliable markers of the epileptogenic zone and surgical outcome [126].

Focal interictal regional hypometabolism can predict good surgical outcome [107, 127–129]. Additionally, extent of resection of PET abnormalities is found to correlate with post operative outcome [130]. Bilateral temporal hypometabolism is associated with a less optimistic surgical outcome and in 50% of patients reflects bilateral foci [131]. Patients with focal temporal abnormalities have more than 90% likelihood of good surgical outcome, and in those without, this figure is reduced to about 63% [128, 129]. The ability to confirm the focus and predict surgical outcome is better when quantitative means are used, typically when asymmetry indexes [AI; e.g., AI = 2(left − right)/(left + right)] are greater than two standard deviations from normative data. Cortical segmentation may also improve yield for FDG-PET but not SPECT [132]. Focal abnormalities on [18F]FDG-PET may reduce the need for or extent of, invasive monitoring [104, 128, 129]. Nonetheless, questions of frontal versus temporal focus may not always reliably be resolved by interictal [18F]FDG-PET studies, and invasive studies or other PET ligand studies may be needed. Conflicting localizing or lateralization data nearly always merit invasive monitoring. False lateralization by PET has been demonstrated after surgery [103], specifically when interpretation relied upon non-quantitative analysis, or occurred during subclinical seizures [103, 133, 134].

[18F]FDG-PET is less efficacious in identifying the epileptogenic zone in extratemporal lobe epilepsy [135]. Most extratemporal lobe epilepsy series include patients with structural lesions that show concordant hypometabolism. When patients with abnormal MRI findings are excluded, 11–50% of the relatively small patient populations remaining show regional decreases in glucose consumption [109, 126]. FDG-PET abnormalities remote from the lesion lessen prospects of good surgical outcome. Abnormal focal PET (or SPECT) findings should be followed by review of "normal" MRI, as focal MRI findings often ensue and will positively affect yield of epilepsy surgery [136–138].

In absence seizures, glucose consumption and perfusion are globally increased [139]. [15O]Water studies performed during electroencephalographic (EEG) bursts of spike and wave demonstrate not only an increase in global perfusion but also a preferential increase in the thalamic regions, supporting the notion of the thalamus as the facilitator of absence events [140]. Interestingly, there is some evidence that valproate decreases cerebral blood flow in the thalamus, which may explain the effect of valproate in controlling generalized epilepsies. In Juvenile myoclonic epilepsy, [(11)C]PE2I, a marker of dopamine transporter (DAT) activity is reduced in midbrain and the high-affinity dopamine (D2/D3) receptor ligand [18F]Fallypride ([(18) F]FP) is reduced in putamen [141].

Some children with a generalized EEG and normal MRI can exhibit regional metabolic abnormalities [142]. "Interictal" FDG-PET will show hypermetabolic areas in

2–6% of pediatric studies. Regional uptake is associated with frequent spike activity and originates from focal cortical dysplasia. Intracranial EEG finds these regions are effectively in status and, when resected, are associated with good outcome [143, 144]. In some children, however, the metabolic abnormalities seen at onset of infantile spasms may resolve or shift with time and thus may represent a functional state that is potentially reversible with successful medical therapy [145, 146]. In children with Rasmussen's encephalitis and hemimegalencephaly, widespread hemispheric hypometabolism is typically seen. PET has been advocated in some circumstances to assess the integrity of the good hemisphere before extensive cortical resection [116, 147]. Isolated hemispheric abnormalities are associated with excellent outcomes for hemispherectomy (90%) but contralateral abnormalities may also be associated with good outcomes (75%) [148]. In tuberous sclerosis, tubers are often hypometabolic, whereas there is some evidence that the more epileptogenic tubers have increased serotonin or kynurenic acid synthesis, reflected by increased [11C]AMT uptake [149, 150]. [11C]AMT uptake is also increased in focal cortical dysplasia when MRI (especially in children <2 years) and [18F]FDG-PET may be normal [149–151]. In hypothalamic hamartoma, remote frontal and parietal cortical hypometabolism appears to be associated with cognitive impairment [152].

### 3.2 SPECT

SPECT ligands used in epilepsy are primarily markers of perfusion, though some receptor ligands are also available, such as [123I]iomazenil ([123I]IMZ) for benzodiazepine receptor studies. The compounds that mark blood flow, HMPAO and ECD, have a distribution in the brain that is proportional to cerebral blood flow. Both ligands are lipophilic; they readily cross the blood-brain barrier on their first pass through brain tissue, become trapped, and exhibit little subsequent redistribution. A potential limitation is that neither ligand has linear uptake at high cerebral blood flow rates, and thus, cerebral blood flow is underestimated under certain circumstances [153]. The efficacy of HMPAO and ECD in epilepsy studies is comparable.

For an ictal SPECT study to be useful, injection of the ligand must occur no later than 30 seconds after cessation of the seizure. The earlier the injection (<20 seconds from seizure onset), the more reliable are the study results [154, 155]; injections after 20 seconds will result in image propagation from the seizure onset zone and lessen localization value [156, 157]. SPECT ligands have a longer half-life compared to PET. 99mTc-Hexamethyl-propyleneamine oxime (99mTc-HMPAO) or 99mTc-ethyl cysteinate dimer (99mTc-ECD) for cerebral perfusion has replaced 123I-based ligands such as [123I]iodoamphetamine and [123I]trimethyl-hydroxymethyl-iodobenzylpropane diamine, because these ligands have a rapid first-pass uptake and long half-life. The long half-life permits bedside injection at ictus and offers a longer window of injectability (from 30 minutes to 4 hours after composition) as well as time to arrange for data acquisition scanning within 4–6 hours after injection. During ictus, there is focal increase in cerebral blood flow to involved cortex, often with decreased perfusion in adjacent areas. After the seizure, there is postictal hypoperfusion, which may return to an interictal state rapidly [158]. Postictal hypoperfusion abnormalities are more reliable than interictal hypoperfusion (60–70% vs. 40–50%, respectively). After ligand injection, lorazepam is sometimes administered to diminish the likelihood of subsequent seizures. It is important to recall that if a patient has multiple seizure types, each type must be captured. Automated systems may be helpful to improve timing (approximately 8 seconds) and reliability of ligand delivery; video-EEG monitoring is critical for interpretation of SPECT studies [159, 160].

The usefulness of SPECT ictal studies approaches that of [18F]FDG-PET in patients with TLE, and ictal studies are probably superior for extratemporal focus localization [161–163]. Partial seizures often show more reliable results than secondarily generalized seizures [164]. False localization is reported in 3–4% of studies, presumably because of seizure propagation, and is more likely to occur with later injection times [107]. Subtraction techniques with MRI co-registration provide enhanced comparison and semiquantitation of perfusion changes between the interictal and ictal states compared with visual comparison alone. Focal ictal SPECT can also predict whether surgical outcome will be good. SPECT is considered most useful in evaluating patients with nonlesional partial epilepsy, especially extra-temporal partial epilepsy. Ictal subtraction SPECT may also be useful in evaluating patients who have failed initial surgery.

Interictal SPECT studies demonstrate regional hypoperfusion in 40–50% of patients with partial epilepsy of temporal lobe origin. However, approximately 5–10% of studies are falsely lateralizing [106, 107, 109, 165, 166].

## 4. Neuroimaging and brain connectome

To date, structural connectivity analyses have been able to demonstrate abnormal networks in patients with epilepsy. There is decreased fiber density of connections in the limbic system among patients with medial TLE [130], which is paradoxically associated with increased nodal clustering and efficiency in the thalamus, insula, and superior temporal regions [131]. Other studies have further revealed atypically strong thalamic–limbic connections with aberrant linkages beyond the medial temporal lobes [167]. These atypical patterns of simultaneous brain activity appear to translate to a reorganization of the functional connectome [168–176]. Reorganization of the functional connectome in epilepsy also appears to be confounded by age [177], age of seizure onset [173, 178], and disease duration [179], reflecting the importance of understanding how disease burden can affect atypical functional patterns.

Identifying these deviant connectome patterns is important because it helps us understand the abnormal plasticity associated with epilepsy and what architectural changes to the brain network provide the substrate for hyperexcitable states. In addition, there is a potential role for identification of specific aberrant connections that may help phenotype different subgroups according to brain imaging parameters and clinical features. For instance, language difficulties in epilepsy have been associated with altered patterns in functional connectivity involving language areas [180], especially when hippocampal sclerosis occurs in the dominant hemisphere [119].

Connectome-based lesion-symptom mapping (CLSM) is a novel approach to lesion mapping that establishes relationships between behavioral measures and specific white matter tracts in the connectome using statistical methods [151]. At the individual level this has the potential to predict clinical outcomes and guide tailored treatments on a case-by-case basis [106, 149]. With approximately one-third of patients with seizures refractory to multiple antiseizure medications [181], and with epilepsy surgery now considered an effective treatment for drug-resistant focal epilepsy [182], it is paramount to identify the factors that may affect postoperative seizure control. Clinical variables alone, however, have been insufficient to predict postoperative outcome. This points to the direction that epilepsy is more of a network disorder than a purely lesional one. It is in this context that network imaging may help to more accurately predict which patients are likely to benefit from epilepsy surgery.

Nowadays computational algorithm based on machine learning is capable of classifying patients who become seizure free postsurgically by analyzing fiber density values with an accuracy of 70% [144]. White matter tracts including the fimbria-fornix, the uncinate fasciculus, and the parahippocampal white matter bundle, have been suggested to contribute to seizure propagation. Reorganization of structural networks after surgery can affect seizure control outcomes [138]. Each patient exhibits different network patterns at the individual level. Features located in the contralateral hemisphere can contribute to prediction accuracy. Deep learning has been shown to be able to sieve through connectivity information derived from presurgical MRI of patients to identify biomarkers which can predict surgical outcome [183]. For example, in TLE patients with persistent postoperative seizures, circumscribed alterations in two regions were found in those with poor postoperative seizure control: the dorsal segment of the ipsilateral fornix and the contralateral parahippocampal white matter bundle [141].

In addition to predicting outcome, network imaging may prove useful in planning surgical targets. Utilization of diffusion measures to study white matter tracts can yield information on laterality of the lesion [184]. While promising, it is important to note that the aforesaid findings were all yielded from retrospective analyses and must therefore be validated in prospective studies.

## 5. Outlook for clinical translation: what lies ahead in the field of connectomics and epilepsy?

The vast amount of data generated by neuroimaging makes it a good candidate for computational methodological analysis. This has shed light on epilepsy as a disease of brain networks. While connectome-derived data have been instrumental thus far in improving and expanding our understanding of the pathophysiology of seizure propagation in difficult-to-treat epilepsy. The generation of personalized connectome is clearly the next step forward in presurgical epilepsy workup in the era of personalized medicine. In doing so our understanding of the brain network will be further expanded benefiting not only epilepsy patients but other neurological and neurosurgical patients alike.

## 6. Conclusions

Improving noninvasive localization is paramount in the surgical treatment of refractory epilepsies. MRI postprocessing techniques allow for more accurate identification of epileptogenic abnormalities, and in doing so they have the potential to increase the diagnostic yield, reduce the need for invasive electrophysiological investigations, and improve epilepsy surgical outcome in years to come. Patient centered connectome-based lesion-symptom mapping will be the future for epilepsy management where therapeutic options can be tailored in order to enable best informed management for both clinicians and patients in their lifelong journey with this disease.

## Author details

Lau Sau Ning Sarah*, Cheng King Fai Kevin and Grace Ho
Queen Mary Hospital, Hong Kong, China

*Address all correspondence to: lsn617@ha.org.hk

## References

[1] Penfield W, Jasper H. Epilepsy and the Functional Anatomy of the Human Brain. Little, Brown and Company: Boston, MA; 1954

[2] Rosenow F, Luders H. Presurgical evaluation of epilepsy. Brain. 2001;**124**(Pt 9):1683-1700

[3] Wyllie E, Lachhwani DK, Gupta A, et al. Successful surgery for epilepsy due to early brain lesions despite generalized EEG findings. Neurology. 2007;**69**(4):389-397

[4] Phal PM, Usmanov A, Nesbit GM, et al. Qualitative comparison of 3-T and 1.5-T MRI in the evaluation of epilepsy. AJR. American Journal of Roentgenology. 2008;**191**(3):890-895

[5] Strandberg M, Larsson EM, Backman S, et al. Pre-surgical epilepsy evaluation using 3T MRI. Do surface coils provide additional information? Epileptic Disorders. 2008;**10**(2):83-92

[6] Knake S, Triantafyllou C, Wald LL, et al. 3T phased array MRI improves the presurgical evaluation in focal epilepsies: A prospective study. Neurology. 2005;**65**(7):1026-1031

[7] Winston GP, Micallef C, Kendell BE, et al. The value of repeat neuroimaging for epilepsy at a tertiary referral center: 16 years of experience. Epilepsy Research. 2013;**105**:349-355

[8] Schmitz BL, Aschoff AJ, Hoffmann MH, et al. Advantages and pitfalls in 3T MR brain imaging: A pictorial review. American Journal of Neuroradiology. 2005;**26**(9):2229-2237

[9] Schmitz BL, Gron G, Brausewetter F, et al. Enhancing gray-to-white matter contrast in 3T T1 spin-echo brain scans by optimizing flip angle. American Journal of Neuroradiology. 2005;**26**(8):2000-2004

[10] Lee SK, Yun CH, Oh JB, et al. Intracranial ictal onset zone in nonlesional lateral temporal lobe epilepsy on scalp ictal EEG. Neurology. 2003;**23**:757-764

[11] Andermann F. Pseudotemporal vs neocortical temporal epilepsy: Things aren't always where they seem to be. Neurology. 2003;**61**:732-733

[12] Tassi L, Colombo N, Garbelli R, et al. Focal cortical dysplasia: Neuropathological subtypes, EEG, neuroimaging and surgical outcome. Brain. 2002;**125**(Pt 8):1719-1732

[13] Colombo N, Tassi L, Galli C, et al. Focal cortical dysplasias: MR imaging, histopathologic, and clinical correlations in surgically treated patients with epilepsy. American Journal of Neuroradiology. 2003;**24**(4):724-733

[14] Ruggieri PM, Najm I, Bronen R, et al. Neuroimaging of the cortical dysplasias. Neurology. 2004;**62**(6 Suppl. 3):S27-S29

[15] Sankar R, Curran JG, Kevill JW, et al. Microscopic cortical dysplasia in infantile spasms: Evolution of white matter abnormalities. American Journal of Neuroradiology. 1995;**16**(6):1265-1272

[16] Eltze CM, Chong WK, Bhate S, et al. Taylor-type focal cortical dysplasia in infants: Some MRI lesions almost disappear with maturation of myelination. Epilepsia. 2005;**46**(12):1988-1992

[17] Hu J, Yu Y, Juhasz C, et al. MR susceptibility weighted imaging (SWI) complements conventional contrast enhanced T1 weighted MRI in characterizing brain abnormalities of Sturge-Weber syndrome. Journal of Magnetic Resonance Imaging. 2008;**28**(2):300-307

[18] Juhasz C, Haacke EM, Hu J, et al. Multimodality imaging of cortical and white matter abnormalities in Sturge–Weber syndrome. American Journal of Neuroradiology. 2007;**28**(5):900-906

[19] Le Bihan D, Mangin JF, Poupon C, et al. Diffusion tensor imaging: Concepts and applications. Journal of Magnetic Resonance Imaging. 2001;**13**(4):534-546

[20] Nakasu Y, Nakasu S, Kizuki H, et al. Changes in water diffusion of rat limbic system during status epilepticus elicited by kainate. Psychiatry and Clinical Neurosciences. 1995;**49**(3):S228-S230

[21] Nakasu Y, Nakasu S, Morikawa S, et al. Diffusion-weighted MR in experimental sustained seizures elicited with kainic acid. American Journal of Neuroradiology. 1995;**16**(6):1185-1192

[22] Righini A, Pierpaoli C, Alger JR, et al. Brain parenchyma apparent diffusion coefficient alterations associated with experimental complex partial status epilepticus. Magnetic Resonance Imaging. 1994;**12**(6):865-871

[23] Wang Y, Majors A, Najm I, et al. Postictal alteration of sodium content and apparent diffusion coefficient in epileptic rat brain induced by kainic acid. Epilepsia. 1996;**37**(10):1000-1006

[24] Diehl B, Najm I, Ruggieri P, et al. Periictal diffusion-weighted imaging in a case of lesional epilepsy. Epilepsia. 1999;**40**(11):1667-1671

[25] Diehl B, Najm I, Ruggieri P, et al. Postictal diffusion-weighted imaging for the localization of focal epileptic areas in temporal lobe epilepsy. Epilepsia. 2001;**42**(1):21-28

[26] Oh JB, Lee SK, Kim KK, et al. Role of immediate postictal diffusion-weighted MRI in localizing epileptogenic foci of mesial temporal lobe epilepsy and non-lesional neocortical epilepsy. Seizure. 2004;**13**(7):509-516

[27] Hufnagel A, Weber J, Marks S, et al. Brain diffusion after single seizures. Epilepsia. 2003;**44**(1):54-63

[28] Milligan TA, Zamani A, Bromfield E. Frequency and patterns of MRI abnormalities due to status epilepticus. Seizure. 2009;**18**:104-108

[29] Nelles M, Bien CG, Kurthen M, et al. Transient splenium lesions in presurgical epilepsy patients: Incidence and pathogenesis. Neuroradiology. 2006;**48**(7):443-448

[30] Sirin S, Gonul E, Kahraman S, et al. Imaging of posterior fossa epidermoid tumors. Clinical Neurology and Neurosurgery. 2005;**107**(6):461-467

[31] Song SK, Sun SW, Ramsbottom MJ, et al. Dysmyelination revealed through MRI as increased radial (but unchanged axial) diffusion of water. NeuroImage. 2002;**17**(3):1429-1436

[32] Song SK, Sun SW, Ju WK, et al. Diffusion tensor imaging detects and differentiates axon and myelin degeneration in mouse optic nerve after retinal ischemia. NeuroImage. 2003;**20**(3):1714-1722

[33] Song SK, Yoshino J, Le TQ, et al. Demyelination increases radial diffusivity in corpus callosum of mouse brain. NeuroImage. 2005;**26**(1):132-140

[34] Beaulieu C, Does MD, Snyder RE, et al. Changes in water diffusion due to Wallerian degeneration in peripheral nerve. Magnetic Resonance in Medicine. 1996;**36**(4):627-631

[35] Diehl B, Luders HO. Temporal lobe epilepsy: When are invasive recordings needed? Epilepsia. 2000;**41**(Suppl. 3): S61-S74

[36] Nimsky C, Ganslandt O, Fahlbusch R. Implementation of fiber tract navigation. Neurosurgery. 2007;**61**(Suppl. 1):306-317

[37] Wu JS, Zhou LF, Tang WJ, et al. Clinical evaluation and follow-up outcome of diffusion tensor imaging-based functional neuronavigation: A prospective, controlled study in patients with gliomas involving pyramidal tracts. Neurosurgery. 2007;**61**(5):935-948

[38] Nimsky C, Grummich P, Sorensen AG, et al. Visualization of the pyramidal tract in glioma surgery by integrating diffusion tensor imaging in functional neuronavigation. Zentralblatt für Neurochirurgie. 2005;**66**(3):133-141

[39] Nimsky C, Ganslandt O, Hastreiter P, et al. Preoperative and intraoperative diffusion tensor imaging-based fiber tracking in glioma surgery. Neurosurgery. 2007;**61**(Suppl. 1):178-185

[40] Chen X, Weigel D, Ganslandt O, et al. Diffusion tensor-based fiber tracking and intraoperative neuronavigation for the resection of a brainstem cavernous angioma. Surgical Neurology. 2007;**68**(3):285-291

[41] Salek-Haddadi A, Friston KJ, Lemieux L, et al. Studying spontaneous EEG activity with fMRI. Brain Research Reviews. 2003;**43**(1):110-133

[42] Marques JP, Kober T, Krueger G, et al. MP2RAGE, a self bias-field corrected sequence for improved segmentation and T1-mapping at high field. NeuroImage. 2010;**49**(2):1271-1281

[43] Wisse LEM, Kuijf HJ, Honingh AM, et al. Automated hippocampal subfield segmentation at 7T MRI. American Journal of Neuroradiology. 2016;**37**(6):1050-1057

[44] Henry TR, Chupin M, Lehéricy S, et al. Hippocampal sclerosis in temporal lobe epilepsy: Findings at 7 T. Radiology. 2011;**261**(1):199-209

[45] Santyr BG, Goubran M, Lau JC, et al. Investigation of hippocampal substructures in focal temporal lobe epilepsy with and without hippocampal sclerosis at 7T. Journal of Magnetic Resonance Imaging. 2017;**45**(5):1359-1370. DOI: 10.1002/jmri.25447

[46] Obusez EC, Lowe M, Oh SH, et al. 7T MR of intracranial pathology: Preliminary observations and comparisons to 3T and 1.5T. NeuroImage. 2018;**168**:459-476

[47] Feldman RE, Rutland JW, Fields MC, et al. Quantification of perivascular spaces at 7 T: A potential MRI biomarker for epilepsy. Seizure. 2018;**54**:11-18

[48] Springer E, Dymerska B, Cardoso PL, et al. Comparison of routine brain imaging at 3 T and 7 T. Investigative Radiology. 2016;**51**(8):469-482

[49] Veersema TJ, van Eijsden P, Gosselaar PH, et al. 7 tesla T2*-weighted MRI as a tool to improve detection of focal cortical dysplasia. Epileptic Disorders. 2016;**18**(3):315-323

[50] Veersema TJ, Ferrier CH, Van Eijsden P, et al. Seven tesla MRI improves detection of focal cortical dysplasia in patients with refractory focal epilepsy. Epilepsia Open. 2017;**2**(2):162-171. DOI: 10.1002/epi4.12041

[51] De Ciantis A, Barba C, Tassi L, et al. 7T MRI in focal epilepsy with unrevealing conventional field strength imaging. Epilepsia. 2016;**3**(57):445-454

[52] Colon AJ, van Osch MJP, Buijs M, et al. Detection superiority of 7 T MRI protocol in patients with epilepsy and suspected focal cortical dysplasia. Acta Neurologica Belgica. 2016;**116**(3):259-269

[53] Farid N, Girard HM, Kemmotsu N, et al. Temporal lobe epilepsy: Quantitative MR volumetry in detection of hippocampal atrophy. Radiology. 2012;**264**(2):542-550

[54] Bien CG, Szinay M, Wagner J, et al. Characteristics and surgical outcomes of patients with refractory magnetic resonance imaging–negative epilepsies. Archives of Neurology. 2009;**66**(12):1491-1499

[55] Jeha LE, Najm I, Bingaman W, et al. Surgical outcome and prognostic factors of frontal lobe epilepsy surgery. Brain. 2007;**130**(Pt 2):574-584

[56] Tellez-Zenteno JF, Hernandez Ronquillo L, Moien-Afshari F, et al. Surgical outcomes in lesional and non-lesional epilepsy: A systematic review and meta-analysis. Epilepsy Research. 2010;**89**(2-3):310-318

[57] Bastos AC, Korah IP, Cendes F, et al. Curvilinear reconstruction of 3D magnetic resonance imaging in patients with partial epilepsy: A pilot study. Magnetic Resonance Imaging. 1995;**13**(8):1107-1112

[58] Bastos AC, Comeau RM, Andermann F, et al. Diagnosis of subtle focal dysplastic lesions: Curvilinear reformatting from three-dimensional magnetic resonance imaging. Annals of Neurology. 1999;**46**(1):88-94

[59] Montenegro MA, Li LM, Guerreiro MM, et al. Focal cortical dysplasia: Improving diagnosis and localization with magnetic resonance imaging multiplanar and curvilinear reconstruction. Journal of Neuroimaging. 2002;**12**(3):224-230

[60] Collins DL, Neelin P, Peters TM, et al. Automatic 3D intersubject registration of MR volumetric data in standardized Talairach space. Journal of Computer Assisted Tomography. 1994;**18**(2):192-205

[61] Salmond CH. Distributional assumptions in voxel-based morphometry. NeuroImage. 2002;**17**:1027-1030. DOI: 10.1016/S1053-8119(02)91153-5

[62] Focke NK, Symms MR, Burdett JL, et al. Voxel-based analysis of whole brain FLAR at 3T detects focal cortical dysplasia. Epilepsia. 2008;**49**(5):786-793

[63] Colliot O, Bernasconi N, Khalili N, et al. Individual voxel-based analysis of gray matter in focal cortical dysplasia. NeuroImage. 2006;**29**(1):162-171

[64] Bonilha L, Montenegro MA, Rorden C, et al. Voxel-based morphometry reveals excess gray matter concentration in patients with focal cortical dysplasia. Epilepsia. 2006;**47**(5):908-915

[65] Bruggemann JM, Wilke M, Som SS, et al. Voxel-based morphometry in the detection of dysplasia and neoplasia in childhood epilepsy: Combined grey/white matter analysis augments detection. Epilepsy Research. 2007;**77**:93-101

[66] Salmenpera TM, Symms MR, Rugg-Gunn FJ, et al. Evaluation of quantitative magnetic resonance imaging contrasts in MRI-negative

refractory focal epilepsy. Epilepsia. 2007;**48**(2):229-237

[67] Najm I, Jehi L, Palmini A, et al. Temporal patterns and mechanisms of epilepsy surgery failure. Epilepsia. 2013;**54**(5):772-782

[68] Thom M. Review: Hippocampal sclerosis in epilepsy: A neuropathology review. Neuropathology and Applied Neurobiology. 2014;**40**(5):520-543

[69] Bernasconi A, Bernasconi N, Bernhardt BC, et al. Advances in MRI for "cryptogenic" epilepsies. Nature Reviews. Neurology. 2011;7(10):99-108

[70] Bernasconi N, Bernasconi A, Caramanos Z, et al. Mesial temporal damage in temporal lobe epilepsy: A volumetric MRI study of the hippocampus, amygdala and parahippocampal region. Brain. 2003;**126**(Pt 2):462-469

[71] Bernasconi N, Bernasconi A, Caramanos Z, et al. Entorhinal cortex atrophy in epilepsy patients exhibiting normal hippocampal volumes. Neurology. 2001;**56**(10):1335-1339

[72] Coan AC, Appenzeller S, Bonilha L, et al. Seizure frequency and lateralization affect progression of atrophy in temporal lobe epilepsy. Neurology. 2009;**73**(11):834-842

[73] Keller SS, Mackay CE, Barrick TR, et al. Voxel-based morphometric comparison of hippocampal and extrahippocampal abnormalities in patients with left and right hippocampal atrophy. NeuroImage. 2002;**16**(1):23-31

[74] Bonilha L, Rorden C, Appenzeller S, et al. Gray matter atrophy associated with duration of temporal lobe epilepsy. NeuroImage. 2006;**32**(3):1070-1079

[75] Keller SS, Baker G, Downes JJ, et al. Quantitative MRI of the prefrontal cortex and executive function in patients with temporal lobe epilepsy. Epilepsy & Behavior. 2009;**15**(2):186-195

[76] Bonilha L, Alessio A, Rorden C, et al. Extrahippocampal gray matter atrophy and memory impairment in patients with medial temporal lobe epilepsy. Human Brain Mapping. 2007;**28**(12):1376-1390

[77] Focke NK, Thompson PJ, Duncan JS. Correlation of cognitive functions with voxel-based morphometry in patients with hippocampal sclerosis. Epilepsy & Behavior. 2008;**12**(3):472-476

[78] Guimarães CA, Bonilha L, Franzon RC, et al. Distribution of regional gray matter abnormalities in a pediatric population with temporal lobe epilepsy and correlation with neuropsychological performance. Epilepsy & Behavior. 2007;**11**(4):558-566

[79] Yasuda CL, Valise C, Saúde AV, et al. Dynamic changes in white and gray matter volume are associated with outcome of surgical treatment in temporal lobe epilepsy. NeuroImage. 2010;**49**(1):71-79

[80] Keller SS, Cresswell P, Denby C, et al. Persistent seizures following left temporal lobe surgery are associated with posterior and bilateral structural and functional brain abnormalities. Epilepsy Research. 2007;**74**(2-3):131-139

[81] Bronen RA, Spencer DD, Fulbright RK. Cerebrospinal fluid cleft with cortical dimple: MR imaging marker for focal cortical dysgenesis. Radiology. 2000;**214**:657-663

[82] Yagishita A, Arai N, Maehara T, et al. Focal cortical dysplasia: Appearance on MR images. Radiology. 1997;**203**(2):553-559

[83] Raymond AA, Fish DR, Sisodiya SM, et al. Abnormalities of gyration, heterotopias, tuberous sclerosis, focal cortical dysplasia, microdysgenesis, dysembryoplastic neuroepithelial tumour and dysgenesis of the archicortex in epilepsy. Clinical, EEG and neuroimaging features in 100 adult patients. Brain. 1995;**118**(Pt 3):629-660

[84] Besson P, Andermann F, Dubeau F, et al. Small focal cortical dysplasia lesions are located at the bottom of a deep sulcus. Brain. 2008;**131**(12):3246-3255. DOI: 10.1093/brain/awn224

[85] Van Essen DC. A tension-based theory of morphogenesis and compact wiring in the central nervous system. Nature. 1997;**385**:313-318. DOI: 10.1038/385313a0

[86] Regis J, Tamura M, Park MC, et al. Subclinical abnormal gyration pattern, a potential anatomic marker of epileptogenic zone in patients with magnetic resonance imaging-negative frontal lobe epilepsy. Neurosurgery. 2011;**69**(1):80-93

[87] Kim H, Mansi T, Bernasconi N. Disentangling hippocampal shape anomalies in epilepsy. Frontiers in Neurology. 2013;**4**:131

[88] Voets NL, Bernhardt BC, Kim H, et al. Increased temporolimbic cortical folding complexity in temporal lobe epilepsy. Neurology. 2011;**76**(2):138-144

[89] Bernhardt BC, Bernasconi N, Concha L, et al. Cortical thickness analysis in temporal lobe epilepsy: Reproducibility and relation to outcome. Neurology. 2010;**74**(22):1776-1784

[90] Caciagli L, Bernasconi A, Wiebe S, et al. A meta-analysis on progressive atrophy in intractable temporal lobe epilepsy: Time is brain? Neurology. 2017;**89**(5):506-516

[91] Baulac M, De Grissac N, Hasboun D, et al. Hippocampal developmental changes in patients with partial epilepsy: Magnetic resonance imaging and clinical aspects. Annals of Neurology. 1998;**44**(2):223-233

[92] Bernasconi N, Kinay D, Andermann F, et al. Analysis of shape and positioning of the hippocampal formation: An MRI study in patients with partial epilepsy and healthy controls. Brain. 2005;**128**(Pt 10):2442-2452

[93] Kim H, Mansi T, Bernasconi N, et al. Surface-based multi-template automated hippocampal segmentation: Application to temporal lobe epilepsy. Medical Image Analysis. 2012;**16**(7):1445-1455

[94] Kulaga-Yoskovitz J, Bernhardt BC, Hong SJ, et al. Multi-contrast submillimetric 3 Tesla hippocampal subfield segmentation protocol and dataset. Scientific Data. 2015;**2**:1-9

[95] Caldairou B, Bernhardt BC, Kulaga-Yoskovitz J, et al. A surface patch-based segmentation method for hippocampal subfields. In: Medical Image Computing and Computer-Assisted Intervention (MICCAI) 19th International Conference Proceedings, Part II [Internet]. Athens, Greece: Springer, Cham; 2016. pp. 379-387. Available from: http://link.springer.com/10.1007/978-3-319-46723-8_44

[96] Woermann FG, Barker GJ, Birnie KD, et al. Regional changes in hippocampal T2 relaxation and volume: A quantitative magnetic resonance imaging study of hippocampal sclerosis. Journal of Neurology, Neurosurgery, and Psychiatry. 1998;**65**:656-664

[97] Namer IJ, Waydelich R, Armspach JP, et al. Contribution of T2 relaxation time mapping in the evaluation of cryptogenic temporal lobe epilepsy. NeuroImage. 1998;7(4 Pt 1):304-313

[98] Van Paesschen W, Sisodiya S, Connelly A, et al. Quantitative hippocampal MRI and intractable temporal lobe epilepsy. Neurology. 1995;**45**(12):2233-2240

[99] Bernasconi A, Bernasconi N, Caramanos Z, et al. T2 relaxometry can lateralize mesial temporal lobe epilepsy in patients with normal MRI. NeuroImage. 2000;**12**(6):739-746

[100] Hong SJ, Bernhardt BC, Caldairou B, et al. Multimodal MRI profiling of focal cortical dysplasia type II. Neurology. 2017;**88**(8):734-742

[101] Lin Y, Fang YHD, Wu G, et al. Quantitative positron emission tomography–guided magnetic resonance imaging postprocessing in magnetic resonance imaging–negative epilepsies. Epilepsia. 2018;**59**(8):1583-1594. DOI: 10.1111/epi.14474

[102] Tan YL, Kim H, Lee S, et al. Quantitative surface analysis of combined MRI and PET enhances detection of focal cortical dysplasias. NeuroImage. 2018;**166**:10-18. DOI: 10.1016/j.neuroimage.2017.10.065

[103] Engel J Jr et al. Pathological findings underlying focal temporal lobe hypometabolism in partial epilepsy. Annals of Neurology. 1982;**12**:518-529

[104] Engel J Jr et al. Presurgical evaluation for partial epilepsy: Relative contributions of chronic depth-electrode recordings versus FDG-PET and scalp-sphenoidal ictal EEG. Neurology. 1990;**40**:1670-1677

[105] Theodore WH, Fishbein D, Dubinsky R. Patterns of cerebral glucose metabolism in patients with partial seizures. Neurology. 1988;**38**:1201-1206

[106] Gaillard WD et al. Interictal metabolism and blood flow are uncoupled in temporal lobe cortex of patients with partial epilepsy. Neurology. 1995;**45**:1841-1848

[107] Ho SS et al. Comparison of ictal SPECT and interictal PET in the presurgical evaluation of temporal lobe epilepsy. Annals of Neurology. 1995;**37**:738-745

[108] Knowlton RC et al. Presurgical multimodality neuroimaging in electroencephalographic lateralized temporal lobe epilepsy. Annals of Neurology. 1997;**42**:829-837

[109] Ryvlin P et al. Clinical utility of flumazenil-PET versus [18F] fluorodeoxyglucose-PET and MRI in refractory partial epilepsy. A prospective study in 100 patients. Brain. 1998;**121**:2067-2081

[110] Savic I et al. Limbic reductions of 5-HT1A receptor binding in human temporal lobe epilepsy. Neurology. 2004;**62**(8):1343-1351

[111] Khan N et al. Thalamic glucose metabolism in temporal love epilepsy measured with 18F-FDG positron emission tomography (PET). Epilepsy Research. 1997;**28**:233-243

[112] Foldvary N et al. Correlation of hippocampal neuronal density and FDG-PET in mesial temporal lobe epilepsy. Epilepsia. 1999;**40**:26-29

[113] Theodore WH et al. Hippocampal volume and glucose metabolism in temporal lobe epileptic foci. Epilepsia. 2001;**42**(1):130-132

[114] O'Brien TJ et al. Hippocampal atrophy is not a major determinant of regional hypometabolism in temporal lobe epilepsy. Epilepsia. 1997;**38**:74-80

[115] Spanaki MV et al. Relationship of seizure frequency to hippocampus volume in temporal lobe epilepsy. Epilepsia. 2000;**41**:1227-1229

[116] Chugani HT et al. Infantile spasms: I. PET identifies focal cortical dysgenesis in cryptogenic cases for surgical treatment. Annals of Neurology. 1990;**27**(4):406-413

[117] Tenney JR et al. Cerebral glucose hypometabolism is associated with mitochondrial dysfunction in patients with intractable epilepsy and cortical dysplasia. Epilepsia. 2014;**55**(9):1415-1422

[118] Spanaki MV et al. Postoperative changes in cerebral metabolism in temporal lobe epilepsy. Archives of Neurology. 2000;**57**(10):1447-1452

[119] Gaillard WD et al. FDG-PET and volumetric MRI in the evaluation of patients with partial epilepsy. Neurology. 1995;**45**(1):123-126

[120] Gaillard WD et al. Prognosis of children with partial epilepsy: MRI and serial 18FDG-PET. Neurology. 2007;**68**(9):655-659

[121] Matheja P et al. Temporal hypometabolism at the onset of cryptogenic temporal lobe epilepsy. European Journal of Nuclear Medicine. 2001;**28**(5):625-632

[122] Benedek K et al. Longitudinal changes in cortical glucose hypometabolism in children with intractable epilepsy. Journal of Child Neurology. 2006;**21**(1):26-31

[123] Breier JI et al. Effects of duration of epilepsy on the uncoupling of metabolism and blood flow in the complex partial seizures. Neurology. 1997;**48**:1047-1053

[124] Gaillard WD et al. Low incidence of abnormal (18)FDG-PET in children with new onset partial epilepsy: A prospective study. Neurology. 2002;**58**:717-722

[125] Kalviainen R et al. Recurrent seizures may cause hippocampal damage in temporal lobe epilepsy. Neurology. 1998;**50**(5):1377-1382

[126] Kim YK et al. (18)F-FDG PET in localization of frontal lobe epilepsy: Comparison of visual and SPM analysis. Journal of Nuclear Medicine. 2002;**43**(9):1167-1174

[127] Manno EM, Sperling MR, Ding X, et al. Predictors of outcome after temporal lobectomy: Positron emission tomography. Neurology. 1994;**44**:2331-2336

[128] Theodore WH et al. PET measurement of cerebral blood flow and temporal lobectomy. Annals of Neurology. 1994;**36**(2):241-244

[129] Theodore WH et al. FDG-positron emission tomography and invasive EEG: Seizure focus detection and surgical outcome. Epilepsia. 1997;**38**(1):81-86

[130] Vinton AB et al. The extent of resection of FDG-PET hypometabolism relates to outcome of temporal lobectomy. Brain. 2007;**130**(Pt 2):548-560

[131] Koutroumanidis M et al. Significance of interictal bilateral temporal hypometabolism in temporal lobe epilepsy. Neurology. 2000;**54**(9):1811-1821

[132] Elkins KC et al. Utility of gray-matter segmentation of ictal-Interictal perfusion SPECT and interictal 18 F-FDG-PET in medically refractory epilepsy. Epilepsy Research. 2017;**130**:93-100

[133] Nagarajan L et al. Contralateral temporal hypometabolism on positron emission tomography in temporal lobe epilepsy. Acta Neurologica Scandinavica. 1996;**93**:81-84

[134] Sperling MR et al. False lateralization of temporal lobe epilepsy with FDG positron emission tomography. Epilepsia. 1995;**36**:722-727

[135] Lee JJ et al. Frontal lobe epilepsy: Clinical characteristics, surgical outcomes and diagnostic modalities. Seizure. 2008;**17**(6):514-523

[136] Salamon N et al. FDG-PET/MRI coregistration improves detection of cortical dysplasia in patients with epilepsy. Neurology. 2008;**71**(20):1594-1601

[137] Jayakar P et al. Diagnostic test utilization in evaluation for respective epilepsy surgery in children. Epilepsia. 2014;**55**(4):507-518

[138] Ding Y et al. 18F-FDG PET and high-resolution MRI co-registration for pre-surgical evaluation of patients with conventional MRI-negative refractory extra-temporal lobe epilepsy. European Journal of Nuclear Medicine and Molecular Imaging. 2018;**45**(9):1567-1572

[139] Theodore WH et al. Positron emission tomography in generalized seizures. Neurology. 1985;**35**:684-690

[140] Prevett MC et al. Demonstration of thalamic activation during typical absence seizures using H2(15)O and PET. Neurology. 1995;**45**:1396-1402

[141] Landvogt C et al. Alteration of dopamine D2/D3 receptor binding in patients with juvenile myoclonic epilepsy. Epilepsia. 2010;**51**(9):1699-1706

[142] Chugani HT, Conti JR. Etiologic classification of infantile spasms in 140 cases: Role of positron emission tomography. Journal of Child Neurology. 1996;**11**(1):44-48

[143] Bansal L et al. PET hypermetabolism in medically resistant childhood epilepsy: Incidence, associations, and surgical outcome. Epilepsia. 2016;**57**(3):436-444

[144] Schur S et al. Significance of FDG-PET hypermetabolism in children with intractable focal epilepsy. Pediatric Neurosurgery. 2018;**53**(3):153-162

[145] Metsahonkala L et al. Focal and global cortical hypometabolism in patients with newly diagnosed infantile spasms. Neurology. 2002;**58**(11):1646-1651

[146] Natsume J et al. PET in infancy predicts long-term outcome during adolescence in cryptogenic West syndrome. American Journal of Neuroradiology. 2014;**35**(8):1580-1585

[147] Chugani HT et al. Surgery for intractable infantile spasms: Neuroimaging perspectives. Epilepsia. 1993;**34**(4):764-771

[148] Traub-Weidinger T et al. Presurgical evaluation of pediatric epilepsy patients prior to hemispherotomy: The prognostic value of 18F-FDG PET. Journal of Neurosurgery. Pediatrics. 2016;**25**(6):683-688

[149] Fedi M et al. alpha-[11C]-Methyl-L-tryptophan PET identifies the epileptogenic tuber and correlates with interictal spike frequency. Epilepsy Research. 2003;**52**(3):203-213

[150] Chugani DC et al. Imaging epileptogenic tubers in children with tuberous sclerosis complex using alpha-[11C]methyl-L-tryptophan positron emission tomography. Annals of Neurology. 1998;**44**:858-866

[151] Juhasz C et al. Alpha-methyl-L-tryptophan PET detects epileptogenic cortex in children with intractable epilepsy. Neurology. 2003;**60**(6):960-968

[152] Wagner K et al. Reduced glucose metabolism in neocortical network nodes remote from hypothalamic hamartomas reflects cognitive impairment. Epilepsia. 2017;**58**:41-49

[153] Asenbaum S et al. Imaging of cerebral blood flow with technetium-99m-HMPAO and technetium-99m-ECD: A comparison. Journal of Nuclear Medicine. 1998;**39**(4):613-618

[154] Shin WC et al. Ictal hyperperfusion patterns according to the progression of temporal lobe seizures. Neurology. 2002;**58**(3):373-380

[155] Lee SK et al. Ictal SPECT in neocortical epilepsies: Clinical usefulness and factors affecting the pattern of hyperperfusion. Neuroradiology. 2006;**48**(9):678-684

[156] Stamoulis C et al. The promise of subtraction ictal SPECT co-registered to MRI for improved seizure localization in pediatric epilepsies: Affecting factors and relationship to the surgical outcome. Epilepsy Research. 2017;**129**:59-66

[157] Ramchuankiat S et al. Impact of injection time on migration of SPECT seizure onset in temporal lobe epilepsy. Conference Proceedings: Annual International Conference of the IEEE Engineering in Medicine and Biology Society. 2017;**2017**:1465-1468

[158] Rowe CC et al. Patterns of postictal cerebral blood flow in temporal lobe epilepsy: Qualitative and quantitative analysis. Neurology. 1991;**41**(7):1096-1103

[159] Crawford A et al. Remote-controlled automatic injection versus manual injection in ictal SPECT of seizure patients: Experience from a children's hospital. Journal of Nuclear Medicine Technology. 2014;**42**(3):161-162

[160] Setoain X et al. Validation of an automatic dose injection system for Ictal SPECT in epilepsy. Journal of Nuclear Medicine. 2012;**53**(2):324-329

[161] Desai A et al. Interictal PET and ictal subtraction SPECT: Sensitivity in the detection of seizure foci in patients with medically intractable epilepsy: Interictal PET and Ictal Subtraction SPECT. Epilepsia. 2013;**54**(2):341-350

[162] Knowlton RC et al. Functional imaging: II. Prediction of epilepsy surgery outcome. Annals of Neurology. 2008;**64**(1):35-41

[163] von Oertzen TJ et al. Prospective use of subtraction ictal SPECT coregistered to MRI (SISCOM) in presurgical evaluation of epilepsy. Epilepsia. 2011;**52**(12):2239-2248

[164] Varghese GI et al. Clinical use of ictal SPECT in secondarily generalized tonic-clonic seizures. Brain. 2009;**132** (Pt 8):2102-2113

[165] Rowe CC, Berkovic SF, Sia ST. Localization of epileptic foci with postictal single photon emission computed tomography. Annals of Neurology. 1989;**26**:660-668

[166] Markand ON et al. Comparative study of interictal PET and ictal SPECT in complex partial seizures.

Acta Neurologica Scandinavica. 1997;**95**(3):129-136

[167] Siclari F, Prior JO, Rossetti AO. Ictal cerebral positron emission tomography (PET) in focal status epilepticus. Epilepsy Research. 2013;**105**(3):356-361

[168] Henry TR et al. In vivo cerebral metabolism and central benzodiazepine-receptor binding in temporal lobe epilepsy. Neurology. 1993;**43**:1998-2006

[169] Koepp MJ et al. Cerebral benzodiazepine receptors in hippocampal sclerosis. An objective in vivo analysis. Brain. 1996;**119**:1677-1687

[170] Koepp MJ et al. In vivo [11C] flumazenil-PET correlates with ex vivo [3H]flumazenil autoradiography in hippocampal sclerosis. Annals of Neurology. 1998;**43**:618-626

[171] Hammers A et al. Neocortical abnormalities of [11C]-flumazenil PET in mesial temporal lobe epilepsy. Neurology. 2001;**56**(7):897-906

[172] Tanaka S, Yonekura Y, Ikeda A. Presurgical identification of epileptic foci with iodine-123 iomazenil SPECT: Comparison with brain perfusion SPECT and FDG-PET. European Journal of Nuclear Medicine. 1997;**24**:27-34

[173] Fujitani S et al. Statistical parametric mapping of interictal 123I-iomazenil SPECT in temporal lobe epilepsy surgery. Epilepsy Research. 2013;**106**(1-2):173-180

[174] Toczek MT et al. PET imaging of 5-HT1A receptor binding in patients with temporal lobe epilepsy. Neurology. 2003;**60**(5):749-756

[175] Giovacchini G et al. 5-HT 1A receptors are reduced in temporal lobe epilepsy after partial-volume correction. Journal of Nuclear Medicine. 2005;**46**(7):1128-1135

[176] Didelot A et al. PET imaging of brain 5-HT1A receptors in the preoperative evaluation of temporal lobe epilepsy. Brain. 2008;**131**(Pt 10): 2751-2764

[177] Merlet I et al. 5-HT1A receptor binding and intracerebral activity in temporal lobe epilepsy: An [18F] MPPF-PET study. Brain. 2004;**127**(Pt 4): 900-913

[178] Theodore WH et al. PET of serotonin 1A receptors and cerebral glucose metabolism for temporal lobectomy. Journal of Nuclear Medicine. 2012;**53**(9):1375-1382

[179] Natsume J et al. Alpha-[11C] methyl-L-tryptophan and glucose metabolism in patients with temporal lobe epilepsy. Neurology. 2003;**60**(5):756-761

[180] Hajek M et al. Mesiobasal versus lateral temporal lobe epilepsy: Metabolic differences in the temporal lobe shown by interictal; 18F-FDG positron emission tomography. Neurology. 1993;**43**:79-86

[181] Theodore WH et al. Reduced hippocampal 5HT1A PET receptor binding and depression in temporal lobe epilepsy. Epilepsia. 2007;**48**(8):1526-1530

[182] Hirvonen J et al. Increased in vivo expression of an inflammatory marker in temporal lobe epilepsy. Journal of Nuclear Medicine. 2012;**53**(2):234-240

[183] Muzik O et al. Intracranial EEG versus flumazenil and glucose PET in children with extratemporal lobe epilepsy. Neurology. 2000;**54**(1):171-179

[184] Hammers A et al. Central benzodiazepine receptors in malformations of cortical development: A quantitative study. Brain. 2001;**124** (Pt 8):1555-1565

Chapter 3

# Perspective Chapter: Functional Human Brain Connectome in Deep Brain Stimulation (DBS) for Parkinson's Disease (PD)

*Germaine Hiu-Fai Chan*

## Abstract

Historically, the success of DBS depends on the accuracy of electrode localization in neuroanatomical structures. With time, diffusion-weighted magnetic resonance imaging (MRI) and functional MRI have been introduced to study the structural connectivity and functional connectivity in patients with neurodegenerative disorders such as PD. Unlike the traditional lesion-based stimulation theory, this new network stimulation theory suggested that stimulation of specific brain circuits can modulate the pathological network and restore it to its physiological state, hence causing normalization of human brain connectome in PD patients. In this review, we discuss the feasibility of network-based stimulation and the use of connectomic DBS in PD.

**Keywords:** connectome, deep brain stimulation, Parkinson's disease, human connectome project (HCP), human connectome mapping

## 1. Introduction

Parkinson's disease (PD) is the second commonest neurodegenerative disease affecting both motor and non-motor domains [1]. It affects 1 to 2% of persons over the age of 60 years [2]. At present, no treatment is available to stop or slow down disease progression. However, currently available therapies can offer symptomatic relief to the patients [1]. In general, with the use of oral dopaminergic treatment, their symptoms can be controlled for a few years after symptom onset before developing motor and non-motor complications [1, 3]. Device-aided therapies, especially deep brain stimulation (DBS), have been used in the management of advanced PD when oral pharmacological treatment is no longer sufficient to control the symptoms or when the patients cannot tolerate the drugs [4–9].

The success of DBS surgery depends on appropriate candidate selection, accuracy of localization of electrodes and optimal DBS programming and medication titration [10, 11]. Okun et al. reported that 46% of patients with referred DBS failure were found to have suboptimal lead placement. Among these patients with lead misplacement, 52% improved with lead replacement [10]. This highlights the importance of precise electrode localization in DBS surgery.

Historically, subthalamic nucleus (STN) and globus pallidus internus (GPi) are common surgical targets in PD patients undergoing DBS surgery [12–18]. Although neurostimulation at these surgical targets can improve motor function and may lead to a reduction in dopaminergic medication dosage, a few issues have been reported with the implantation of neurostimulators at STN and GPi. First, these surgical targets such as STN, though small, were found to be divided into functional subzones [19–21]. Therefore, even with precise electrode localization, patients undergoing DBS surgeries can develop neuropsychiatric complications. Lambert et al. showed that the STN was divided into 3 functional subzones (anterior: "limbic" subzone; middle: "associative" subzone; posterior: "motor" subzone) with the use of diffusion weighted imaging (DWI) [19]. Ewert et al. revealed that the GPi can divided into 7 subzones (motor, premotor, sensory, prefrontal, posterior parietal, temporal and occipital), of which motor, premotor and sensory subzones are grouped together as the sensorimotor functional zone and lie in the posterior third of the GPi [21]. Second, these surgical targets are small and close to other salient anatomical structures in the brain. Let us take the STN as an example. The STN is small ($12 \times 5 \times 3$ mm$^3$) and lies next to structures such as internal capsule, medial lemniscus, corticospinal tract, and red nucleus. With suboptimal electrode placement or overstimulation, electrical current can be spread to these adjacent structures, resulting in side effects (**Table 1**) [22]. Third, even though STN and GPi are known to be effective targets in relieving PD symptoms, different symptom may have small difference in the site for effective neurostimulation [23]. On the contrary, lesions from different brain locations can result in similar symptoms [24]. Therefore, PD DBS surgeries at these conventional surgical targets, even if the localization is accurate, can vary in treatment response. Furthermore, a PD patient may have more than one symptom, either motor or non-motor symptom, and so neurostimulation at one surgical target may not be sufficient to alleviate his symptoms.

| Electrode location / Direction of current spread | Anatomical structures affected | Clinical effects |
|---|---|---|
| STN DBS | | |
| Optimal location | STN | Dyskinesia |
| Too inferior / medial | Oculomotor fibers | Diplopia |
| Too posterior / medial | Medial lemniscus | Paraesthesia |
| Too anterior / lateral | Internal capsule<br>Corticospinal fibers | Tonic muscle contraction |
| Too anterior / lateral | Internal capsule<br>Corticobulbar fibers | Dysarthria |
| Too inferior | Cerebellothalamic tract | Ataxia |
| Too inferior | Substantia nigra | Mood changes |
| GPi DBS | | |
| Too posterior / medial | Internal capsule | Tonic muscle contraction |
| Too posterior / medial | Internal capsule<br>Corticobulbar fibers | Dysarthria |
| Too inferior | Optic tract | Visual phenomena |

**Table 1.**
*Side effects of STN / GPi DBS with respect to the anatomy of the surgical targets [22].*

To better control symptoms with DBS surgery, researchers have explored the possibility of better localizing the sites responsible for patients' symptoms and linking these sites together to form a circuit or network. It has been postulated that if a circuit connecting these sites can be mapped out for each patient individually, stimulating the circuit, instead of the traditional way of stimulating the anatomical structure, may be a better therapeutic option.

In this review, we will discuss

- The concept of human connectome
- The concept of normative connectome
- The application of normative connectome in neuromodulation
- Connectomic DBS in PD

## 2. The concept of human connectome

According to the classical teaching, localization of lesions in the nervous system accounts for most of the neurological features. In reality, we found that this approach has some limitations. First, lesion-based localization approach is occasionally unclear. Lesions causing the same symptom can occur in various parts in the brain, whereas one cerebral lesion can result in different neurological symptoms. As a result, the relationship between neurological symptoms and lesion location is not often straightforward [25–27]. Second, it is not uncommon to have patients with complex neurological and psychiatric symptoms unable to find obvious cerebral lesions from neuroimaging [27]. Therefore, it has been speculated that these neurological symptoms, instead of resulting from overt lesions in the nervous system, may be caused by disruption of anatomical and functional networks created by interacting neural elements, which are at a more microscopic level.

To study the human brain network, we have to understand the concept of human connectome. The human connectome is defined as "a comprehensive structural description of the network and connections forming the human brain" [25, 26]. In general, the term "connectome" has three major components.

First, the connectome is a description of structures and studies the set of physical links between neural elements. To examine the connections between neural elements, we need to look at both *structural* and *functional connectivity*.

*Structural connectivity* offers a consistent anatomical description of structural connections within the nervous system. At the micro- and meso-scales, structural connectivity reveals synaptic coupling between cells or long-distance axonal projections between neuronal populations [28, 29]. On the other hand, at the macroscale, structural connectivity points to large, myelinated white matter fiber bundles, which can be visualized with diffusion-weighted MRI data using the tractography software packages [30, 31].

As for *functional connectivity*, it means correlations in activation among spatially distinct brain regions, either in a resting state or with external stimuli, and can be measured as the bivariate correlation of their activities when using functional MRI data [26, 32–34].

Second, the connectome is merely a description of brain connectivity across multiple spatial scales. However, it does not offer all the information of cells and synapses at the microscale level [26].

Thirdly and most importantly, the concept of the connectome is that it is a description of a neural network [26]. With the use of mathematical and statistical approaches, the connectome is an object that fits within a larger theoretical framework, thereby linking neuroscience to network science and complex systems [26].

## 3. Approach to mapping the human connectome

As discussed in last section, the human connectome is a structural description of the neural network and connections across multiple spatial scales. In general, there are three scales of organization within the human brain [26]:

- The microscale of single neurons and synapses [35, 36]
- The mesoscale of neuronal populations and their interconnecting circuitry [37–39]
- The macroscale of anatomically distinct brain regions and pathways

Mapping of the connectome at the first two levels usually occurs in animal models and is conducted in experimental trials. In this review, we will focus on the mapping of the human connectome at the macroscale.

At present, MRI has been used as a non-invasive tool for mapping of large-scale structural connections in the human brain [26, 27]. Both *structural* and *functional connectivity* need to be studied in detail.

*Structural connectivity* is usually assessed by diffusion-weighted MRI sequences, followed by probabilistic tractography, because water moves more freely along white matter fiber bundles than across them and so white matter pathways can be reconstructed, thereby identifying fibers that pass between various brain regions [27].

In contrast, resting state functional MRI (rfMRI) is frequently used to study *functional connectivity*. It examines the blood oxygen level dependent (BOLD) signal, which serves as an indirect marker of neuronal activity [27, 34]. When brain activity increases, blood flow and glucose consumption increase much more than oxygen consumption. Therefore, the amount of deoxygenated hemoglobin decreases in the region of increased activity and the BOLD signal is enhanced [40]. *Functional connectivity* is defined as the statistical association between time-series of anatomically distinct brain regions, which in functional MRI is typically calculated as zero-lag correlation. In other words, if two brain regions have BOLD signals that are correlated, they are functionally connected [34].

With the use of diffusion-weighted MRI and functional MRI, the functional human connectome can be mapped out at the macroscale [25, 27]. The approach to mapping the human connectome is outlined as follows (**Figure 1**) [25].

**Step 1:**

First, diffusion-weighted MRI, followed by probabilistic tractography of thalamocortical tracts and corticocortical interareal pathways, should be performed to aid in the parcellation of the human brain, thereby creating a voxel-wise probabilistic all-to-all *structural connectivity* matrix.

**Step 2:**

Second, a correlation analysis of spatially registered resting state and/or task-based functional MRI recorded in the same person is then accomplished to construct a voxel-wise all-to-all *functional connectivity* matrix for the human brain.

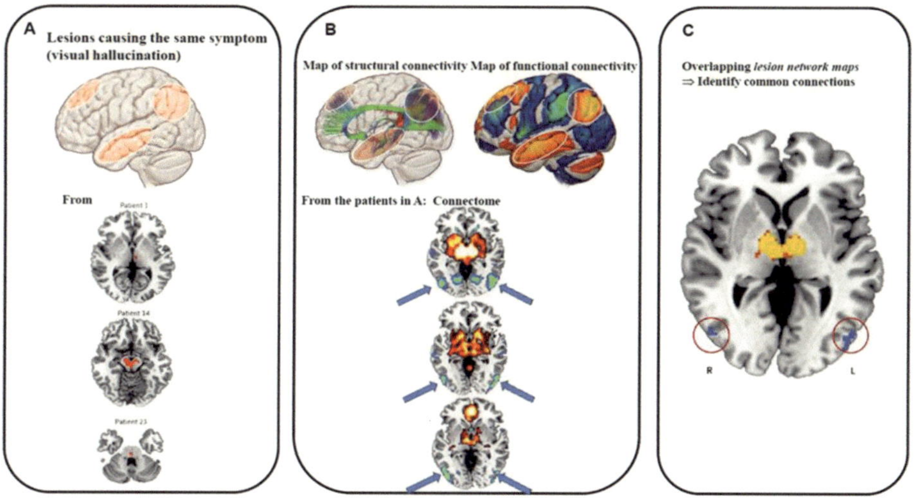


**Figure 1.**
*Using the human brain connectome to localize symptoms [27].*

**Step 3:**

Subsequently, a cluster analysis of correspondences between the structural and functional connectivity matrix obtained from the last two steps is carried out. With that, the human brain regions of consistent structure-function relationships can be found.

In this way, it is possible for us to map out the human connectome. To further improve the quality of the connectome, we may need to compare the mapped network with animal models to look for correspondences and deviations. Also, the predictions generated from the structural-functional connectivity matrix can be validated with specific stimulation techniques.

## 4. Normative connectome and the human connectome project (HCP)

Even though human connectome is a big step in enhancing localization in the nervous system, it is time-consuming, expensive and may be exhausting to the patients because they have to go through a lengthy process of image acquisitions with functional MRI and diffusion-weighted MRI. In fact, in a clinical imaging context, the human connectomes can be studied with either individual MRI data or the MRI data from a group of individuals. The latter approach gives rise to an idea known as a *normative connectome*, which is described as an average or generalized wiring diagram of the human brain [27].

Normative connectome can be useful in those who fail to obtain their own connectomes [27]. For instance, in PD patients with severe tremor or dyskinesia, they may not be able to obtain good-quality MRI images without motion artifacts. Besides, in those patients with cerebral lesions such as cerebrovascular accident, they may not be able to obtain their own connectome even if they can tolerate the long procedure of image acquisition. It is because with previous cerebral insults, that specific region(s) in the brain may have been damaged, thereby disrupting the cerebral circuitry focally and making it impossible to map out the functional connectivity accurately. Nevertheless, normative connectome, which is obtained from group MRI data, cannot provide each individual information of connectivity of his own brain, and may not reflect his actual situation. It can vary with age, gender, body mass index and neurological diseases [41–46].

As such, research studying normative connectome of the human brain has grown in number over the last five to ten years and the Human Connectome Project (HCP) is a good example. It is a large-scale project conducted in the U.S. to examine the human brain circuits and their relationship to behavior in a large population of healthy adults at a macroscopic level [27, 47, 48]. Clinical and neuroimaging information obtained in this project were listed out as follows [47–49].

- Multimodal neuroimaging with 3 T/7 T MRI scanners: structural, functional, and diffusion-weighted MRI
- Magnetoencephalography
- Genetic analyses
- Behavioral assessment

## 5. Applications of normative connectome (including DBS)

As a powerful tool to study the intriguing network in the brain, normative connectome can be used in different areas.

First, normative connectome can unveil the underlying complicated pathways of various neurological and psychiatric diseases and so may bring insights to the identification of new treatment targets. Let us take **Figure 1** as an example. By mapping the connectomes of a group of patients with visual hallucination, lesions that cause the symptom were found to be connected to the occipital cortex. This aid in the discovery of novel treatment targets, as in this example, transcranial magnetic stimulation at the occipital cortex can suppress visual hallucination [50].

Second, normative connectome can enhance surgical precision and hence improve treatment outcome of different neurosurgical procedures. For instance, for glioma patients who plan for resection surgery, the application of normative connectome can help in the identification of eloquent areas and motor tracts before operation, hence reducing the number of intra-operative stimulations required to safely confirm a tract, decreasing the likelihood of disruptive seizures, lowering the risks of post-operative neurological deficits, facilitating the resection, and making patients more comfortable during the operation [51, 52]. Epilepsy surgery is another example. It has been reported that with the use of connectome, the surgical outcome of epilepsy surgery can be improved and the risks of post-operative neurocognitive sequelae, including memory and language impairment, can be reduced [53–56].

Last but not the least, normative connectome has been used widely in the field of neuromodulation, especially DBS. Theoretically, DBS works by depolarization blockade, synaptic inhibition and depression, as well as, stimulation-induced modulation of pathological network activity, of which is regarded the most important mechanism of action [57, 58]. Thus, when normative connectome allows us to map out the pathological pathways in the brain, stimulation at certain points along the circuits may restore the disrupted information flow and so alleviate patients' symptoms. Besides, DBS electrodes, which function as probes, can become *seeds* or regions-of-interest

(ROIs) when they are used to compute their connectivity profiles with normative connectome to perform network-based analyses. In this way, we can identify the optimal site for stimulation and avoid undesirable side effects, thereby facilitating DBS programming and improving surgical outcome [59].

## 6. How to perform connectomic analyses in patients with DBS implanted

Assuming that there is no significant difference between the patient's brain and an average brain, normative connectomic analysis can be conducted to study the patient's connectivity profile that his neurostimulator may modulate. Unlike individual connectomic analysis, either structural or functional MRI data is enough for normative connectomic analysis. In other words, either diffusion-weighted MRI with tractography or functional MRI is required for normative connectomic analysis. With this network analysis, the precision of pre-operative targeting and post-operative programming can be enhanced [23, 60, 61].

The approach to conduct connectomic analysis in a patient with DBS implanted is described as follows (**Figure 2**) [23, 60, 61].

**Step 1: co-registration.**

Before DBS surgery, structural MRI brain, as well as diffusion-weighted or functional MRI brain is performed. After surgery, a computed tomography (CT) of the brain is done. The post-operative CT brain is then co-registered to the pre-operative MRI brain, preferably with brain shift correction and spatial normalization.

**Step 2: electrode localization.**

After co-registration of pre-operative and post-operative neuroimages, the electrodes can be localized while the adjacent neuroanatomical structures are identified.

**Step 3: estimation of volume of tissue activated (VTA).**

The VTA is an estimate of the volume and shape of the distribution of electrical signal stimulating brain tissues when the contact on a DBS electrode is activated. It depends on the composition of settings of the electrode contacts and implanted pulse

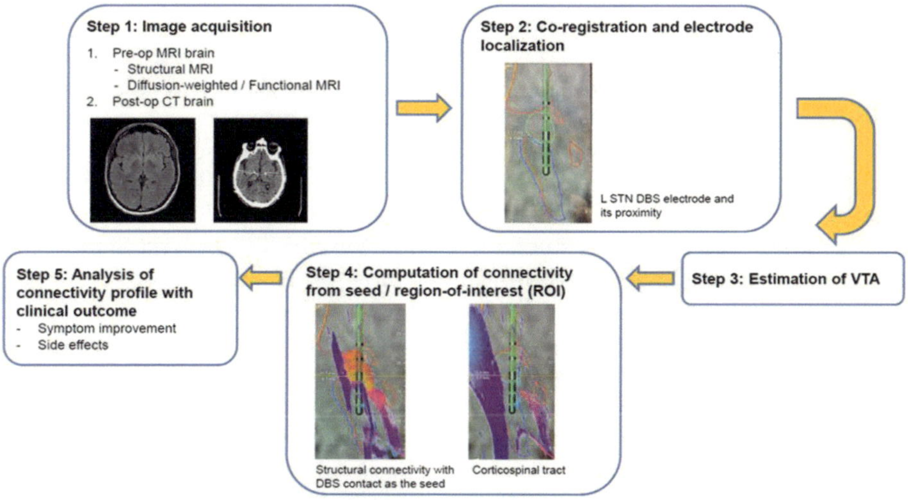


**Figure 2.**
*The approach to perform connectomic analysis in a patient with DBS implanted.*

generator, e.g., the number and locations of activated contacts, impedance, voltage, pulse width, or frequency [62, 63].

After the localization of DBS electrode, the VTA is estimated with the activated contact(s) on the DBS electrode identified. The physician can choose the electrode contact(s) stimulated with monopolar stimulation and decide the stimulation programming setting. The VAT will be estimated according to the DBS programming parameters.

**Step 4: calculation of connectivity profile from seed region.**

When a region-of-interest (ROI) has been identified, it can be used as a seed within specific functional or structural normative connectomes to work out its functional or structural connectivity, respectively. Usually, the VTA of a specific DBS electrode is selected as the seed.

**Step 5: analysis of the relationship of DBS site connectivity with clinical outcome.**

Finally, a statistical analysis is conducted to investigate if there is a relationship between DBS site connectivity and clinical outcome, which can be symptom improvement or side effects.

## 7. Connectomic DBS in PD

Indeed, the use of human connectome has been studied extensively in the field of DBS surgery, especially for major movement disorder indications such as PD. In general, electrode localization is important in the success of surgery. Historically, lesion-based localization at surgical targets, namely STN or GPi, is found to improve motor symptoms in PD patients. However, as increasing evidence points out that DBS works by restoring the connectivity of abnormal networks to a physiological state, [57, 58] more studies have investigated the relationship between connectivity-based localization and treatment outcome of DBS surgery. Horn et al. reported that with the use of normative connectome, structural connectivity to supplementary motor area (SMA), superior frontal gyrus and cerebellum were associated with good clinical response. Also, structural and functional connectivity were independent predictors of clinical improvement of STN DBS [45].

Next, it has been postulated that if different surgical targets would modulate the same circuit in PD patients and affect treatment response. Sobesky et al. showed that based on normative connectome atlas, connectivity profiles seeding from either STN or GPi DBS electrodes were highly similar, suggesting that irrespective of the surgical target, the network modulated by DBS largely overlaps [64]. Moreover, in both groups, functional connectivity to the frontal lobe, especially SMA and adjacent cingulate, middle and inferior temporal gyri, inferior parietal gyri and motor cerebellum were associated with good clinical outcome [64]. Nonetheless, despite the marked similarity in the circuitry modulated by both DBS, the treatment response in the two groups varied. For bradykinesia-rigidity symptoms, connectivity profile was associated with significant improvement and shared considerable similarity in both groups. In contrast, the results for tremor were different, suggesting that the networks modulated by effective neurostimulation at different targets, though similar, may have a small discrepancy [64].

Electrophysiological data has long been used as markers for lesion-based neuromodulation surgeries in PD. For example, local field potential (LFP) can serve as a tool for brain sensing in PD patients with DBS implanted at STN, thereby facilitating DBS programming and medication titration. Increased beta activities were observed in the hypodopaminergic state when the patients suffer from bradykinesia and rigidity and could be suppressed by DBS and dopaminergic medications. On the other hand, increased gamma activities were seen in times of dyskinesia [65–69]. However, in patients with connectivity-based stimulation, will the electrophysiological data correlate with the connectivity profile? Accolla et al. described that beta oscillations were detected in the cerebral circuit projecting from the STN to the motor and premotor cortical areas in PD patients [70]. Besides, Hirschmann et al. reported that with the use of magnetoencephalography (MEG), local field potential (LFP) and electromyogram (EMG), elevated beta coherence was found between M1 and STN in PD patients, which could be suppressed with administration of levodopa [71]. These findings suggested a link between electrophysiology data and connectivity-based stimulation.

As such, connectomic DBS seems to be a reasonable and effective therapeutic option for advanced PD patients. Growing evidence has showed that depending on the symptoms, connectomic DBS can act on different circuits in the brain. In this way, the neuromodulation surgery can affect both motor and non-motor functions (**Table 2**) [23, 45, 61, 72–79].

| Study | DBS target | Number of subjects | Type of connectome | Major findings |
|---|---|---|---|---|
| Motor effects | | | | |
| Horn et al. [23] | STN | 51 | Structural connectivity | VTAs connecting to SMA correlated to clinical motor improvement |
| Treu et al. [61] | STN | 51 | Structural connectivity | VTAs connecting to M1 / S1 negatively correlated with motor outcome. |
| Horn et al. [45] | STN | 95 | • Structural connectivity<br>• Functional connectivity | • VTA structural connectivity with SMA associated with clinical motor improvement<br>• Functional connectivity with M1 associated with clinical motor improvement. |
| Tsuboi et al. [72] | GPi | 16 | • Structural connectivity<br>• Functional connectivity | • Stimulation induced dyskinesia (SID) VTAs significantly associated with higher structural connectivity to the associative cortex and SMA / premotor cortex.<br>• Non-SID VTAs associated with greater connectivity to the primary sensory cortex, cerebellum, subthalamic nucleus, and motor thalamus. |

| Study | DBS target | Number of subjects | Type of connectome | Major findings |
|---|---|---|---|---|
| Lofredi et al. [73] | STN | 17 | Structural connectivity | VTAs connecting to the pre-SMA and inferior frontal gyrus of the right hemisphere correlated with stimulation-induced movement inhibition. |
| de Almeida Marcelino et al. [74] | STN | 20 | Functional connectivity | VTAs connecting to M1 and cerebellar hemispheres correlated with motor learning improvement. |
| Avecillas-Chasin et al. [75] | STN | 43 | Structural connectivity | • Stimulation zones related to rigidity and tremor improvement involved pallidofugal pathway.<br>• Stimulation zones related to bradykinesia improvement involved nigrofugal pathway. |
| Lizarraga et al. [76] | STN | 1 | Structural connectivity | VTAs associated with a greater degree of lateral deviation (Pisa syndrome) associated with increased white matter streamlines. |
| Non-motor effects | | | | |
| Irmen et al. [77] | STN | 116 | Structural connectivity | VTAs connecting to left prefrontal cortex associated with worsening of depressive symptoms. |
| Cury et al. [78] | STN | 32 | Structural connectivity | VTAs connecting to a distributed network of sensory brain regions (prefrontal, insular and cingulate cortex, and postcentral gyrus) inversely correlated with pain intensity improvement. |
| Mosley et al. [79] | STN | 55 | Structural connectivity | VTAs connecting to the prefrontal cortex (especially the orbitofrontal cortex) related to impulsivity |

**Table 2.**
*Clinical effects of connectomic DBS in PD.*

## 8. Conclusion

In conclusion, connectomic DBS, which makes use of circuitry-based stimulation technique rather than lesion-based stimulation technique, has revolutionized the field of neuromodulation surgery. By stimulating patient-specific circuits, this surgery enables us to offer a more precise management approach while avoiding undesirable side effects. In addition, with the advent of normative connectome obtained by grouped data, it simplifies the complicated procedure of connectome mapping, trajectory planning and DBS programming, making it more user-friendly to the neurosurgeons and neurologists. Furthermore, connectomic mapping allows us to map out symptom-specific circuits for each patient individually and check for the overlap of these circuits. In this way, connectomic DBS surgery can be tailormade for each patient and become "bespoke surgery" that can address their own needs.

## Author details

Germaine Hiu-Fai Chan
Department of Medicine, Queen Elizabeth Hospital, Hong Kong

*Address all correspondence to: chf862@ha.org.hk

## References

[1] Kalia LV, Lang AE. Parkinson's disease. Lancet. 2015;**386**(9996):896-912. DOI: 10.1016/S0140-6736(14)61393-3

[2] Tanner CM, Aston DA. Epidemiology of Parkinson's disease and akinetic syndromes. Current Opinion in Neurology. 2000;**13**(4):427-430. DOI: 10.1097/00019052-200008000-00010

[3] Aquino CC, Fox SH. Clinical spectrum of levodopa-induced complications. Movement Disorders. 2015;**30**(1):80-89. DOI: 10.1002/mds.26125

[4] Worth PF. When the going gets tough: How to select patients with Parkinson's disease for advanced therapies. Practical Neurology. 2013;**13**(3):140-152. DOI: 10.1136/practneurol-2012-000463

[5] Volkmann J, Albanese A, Antonini A, Chaudhuri KR, Clarke CE, de Bie RM, et al. Selecting deep brain stimulation or infusion therapies in advanced Parkinson's disease: An evidence-based review. Journal of Neurology. 2013;**260**(11):2701-2714. DOI: 10.1007/s00415-012-6798-6

[6] Williams DR, Evans AH, Fung VSC, Hayes M, Iansek R, Kimber T, et al. Practical approaches to commencing device-assisted therapies for Parkinson disease in Australia. Internal Medicine Journal. 2017;**47**(10):1107-1113. DOI: 10.1111/imj.13398

[7] Moro E, Lang AE. Criteria for deep-brain stimulation in Parkinson's disease: Review and analysis. Expert Review of Neurotherapeutics. 2016;**6**(11):1695-1705. DOI: 10.1586/14737175.6.11.1695

[8] Defer GL, Widner H, Marié RM, Rémy P, Levivier M. Core assessment program for surgical interventional therapies in Parkinson's disease (CAPSIT-PD). Movement Disorders. 1999;**14**(4):572-584. DOI: 10.1002/1531-8257(199907)14:4<572::aid-mds1005>3.0.co;2-c

[9] Munhoz RP, Picillo M, Fox SH, Bruno V, Panisset M, Honey CR, et al. Eligibility criteria for deep brain stimulation in Parkinson's disease, tremor, and dystonia. The Canadian Journal of Neurological Sciences. 2016;**43**(4):462-471. DOI: 10.1017/cjn.2016.35. Epub 2016 May 3

[10] Okun MS, Tagliati M, Pourfar M, Fernandez HH, Rodriguez RL, Alterman RL, et al. Management of referred deep brain stimulation failures: A retrospective analysis from two movement disorders centers. Archives of Neurology. 2005;**62**(8):1250-1255. DOI: 10.1001/archneur.62.8.noc40425. Epub 2005 Jun 13

[11] Limousin P, Foltynie T. Long-term outcomes of deep brain stimulation in Parkinson disease. Nature Reviews. Neurology. 2019;**15**(4):234-242. DOI: 10.1038/s41582-019-0145-9

[12] Deuschl G, Schade-Brittinger C, Krack P, Volkmann J, Schäfer H, Bötzel K. Et al; German Parkinson study group, Neurostimulation section. A randomized trial of deep-brain stimulation for Parkinson's disease. The New England Journal of Medicine. 2006;**355**(9):896-908. DOI: 10.1056/NEJMoa060281

[13] Weaver FM, Follett K, Stern M, Hur K, Harris C, Marks WJ Jr, et al. CSP 468 study group. Bilateral deep brain stimulation vs best medical therapy for patients with advanced Parkinson disease: A randomized controlled

trial. Journal of the American Medical Association. 2009;**301**(1):63-73. DOI: 10.1001/jama.2008.929

[14] Okun MS, Fernandez HH, Wu SS, Kirsch-Darrow L, Bowers D, Bova F, et al. Cognition and mood in Parkinson's disease in subthalamic nucleus versus globus pallidus interna deep brain stimulation: The COMPARE trial. Annals of Neurology. 2009;**65**(5):586-595. DOI: 10.1002/ana.21596

[15] Follett KA, Weaver FM, Stern M, Hur K, Harris CL, Luo P, et al. CSP 468 study group. Pallidal versus subthalamic deep-brain stimulation for Parkinson's disease. The New England Journal of Medicine. 2010;**362**(22):2077-2091. DOI: 10.1056/NEJMoa0907083

[16] Weaver FM, Follett KA, Stern M, Luo P, Harris CL, Hur K, et al. CSP 468 study group. Randomized trial of deep brain stimulation for Parkinson disease: Thirty-six-month outcomes. Neurology. 2012;**79**(1):55-65. DOI: 10.1212/WNL.0b013e31825dcdc1. Epub 2012 Jun 20

[17] Odekerken VJ, van Laar T, Staal MJ, Mosch A, Hoffmann CF, Nijssen PC, et al. Subthalamic nucleus versus globus pallidus bilateral deep brain stimulation for advanced Parkinson's disease (NSTAPS study): A randomised controlled trial. Lancet Neurology. 2013;**12**(1):37-44. DOI: 10.1016/S1474-4422(12)70264-8. Epub 2012 Nov 16

[18] Odekerken VJ, Boel JA, Schmand BA, de Haan RJ, Figee M, van den Munckhof P, et al. NSTAPS study group. GPi vs STN deep brain stimulation for Parkinson disease: Three-year follow-up. Neurology. 2016;**86**(8):755-761. DOI: 10.1212/WNL.0000000000002401. Epub 2016 Jan 27

[19] Lambert C, Zrinzo L, Nagy Z, Lutti A, Hariz M, Foltynie T, et al. Confirmation of functional zones within the human subthalamic nucleus: Patterns of connectivity and sub-parcellation using diffusion weighted imaging. NeuroImage. 2012;**60**(1):83-94. DOI: 10.1016/j.neuroimage.2011.11.082. Epub 2011 Dec 8

[20] Benarroch EE. Subthalamic nucleus and its connections: Anatomic substrate for the network effects of deep brain stimulation. Neurology. 2008;**70**(21):1991-1995. DOI: 10.1212/01.wnl.0000313022.39329.65

[21] Ewert S, Plettig P, Li N, Chakravarty MM, Collins DL, Herrington TM, et al. Toward defining deep brain stimulation targets in MNI space: A subcortical atlas based on multimodal MRI, histology and structural connectivity. NeuroImage. 2018;**170**:271-282. DOI: 10.1016/j.neuroimage.2017.05.015. Epub 2017 May 20

[22] Krack P, Fraix V, Mendes A, Benabid AL, Pollak P. Postoperative management of subthalamic nucleus stimulation for Parkinson's disease. Movement Disorders. 2002;**17**(Suppl. 3):S188-S197. DOI: 10.1002/mds.10163

[23] Horn A, Li N, Dembek TA, Kappel A, Boulay C, Ewert S, et al. Lead-DBS v2: Towards a comprehensive pipeline for deep brain stimulation imaging. NeuroImage. 2019;**184**:293-316. DOI: 10.1016/j.neuroimage.2018.08.068. Epub 2018 Sep 1

[24] Karnath HO, Sperber C, Rorden C. Mapping human brain lesions and their functional consequences. NeuroImage. 2018;**165**:180-189. DOI: 10.1016/j.neuroimage.2017.10.028. Epub 2017 Oct 16

[25] Sporns O, Tononi G, Kötter R. The human connectome: A structural description of the human brain. PLoS Computational Biology. 2005;**1**(4):e42. DOI: 10.1371/journal.pcbi.0010042

[26] Sporns O. The human connectome: A complex network. Annals of the New York Academy of Sciences. 2011;**1224**:109-125. DOI: 10.1111/j.1749-6632.2010.05888.x. Epub 2011 Jan 4

[27] Fox MD. Mapping symptoms to brain networks with the human connectome. The New England Journal of Medicine. 2018;**379**(23):2237-2245. DOI: 10.1056/NEJMra1706158

[28] Oh SW, Harris JA, Ng L, Winslow B, Cain N, Mihalas S, et al. A mesoscale connectome of the mouse brain. Nature. 2014;**508**(7495):207-214. DOI: 10.1038/nature13186. Epub 2014 Apr 2

[29] Markov NT, Ercsey-Ravasz MM, Ribeiro Gomes AR, Lamy C, Magrou L, Vezoli J, et al. A weighted and directed interareal connectivity matrix for macaque cerebral cortex. Cerebral Cortex. 2014;**24**(1):17-36. DOI: 10.1093/cercor/bhs270. Epub 2012 Sep 25

[30] Basser PJ, Pajevic S, Pierpaoli C, Duda J, Aldroubi A. In vivo fiber tractography using DT-MRI data. Magnetic Resonance in Medicine. 2000;**44**(4):625-632. DOI: 10.1002/1522-2594(200010)44:4<625::aid-mrm17>3.0.co;2-o

[31] Daducci A, Gerhard S, Griffa A, Lemkaddem A, Cammoun L, Gigandet X, et al. The connectome mapper: An open-source processing pipeline to map connectomes with MRI. PLoS One. 2012;7(12):e48121. DOI: 10.1371/journal.pone.0048121 Epub 2012 Dec 18

[32] Zhou D, Thompson WK, Siegle G. MATLAB toolbox for functional connectivity. NeuroImage. 2009;**47**(4):1590-1607. DOI: 10.1016/j.neuroimage.2009.05.089. Epub 2009 Jun 8

[33] Smith SM, Miller KL, Salimi-Khorshidi G, Webster M, Beckmann CF, Nichols TE, et al. Network modelling methods for FMRI. NeuroImage. 2011;**54**(2):875-891. DOI: 10.1016/j.neuroimage.2010.08.063. Epub 2010 Sep 15

[34] Pervaiz U, Vidaurre D, Woolrich MW, Smith SM. Optimising network modelling methods for fMRI. NeuroImage. 2020;**211**:116604. DOI: 10.1016/j.neuroimage.2020.116604. Epub 2020 Feb 13

[35] White JG, Southgate E, Thomson JN, Brenner S. The structure of the nervous system of the nematode Caenorhabditis elegans. Philosophical Transactions of the Royal Society of London. Series B, Biological Sciences. 1986;**314**(1165):1-340. DOI: 10.1098/rstb.1986.0056

[36] Chen BL, Hall DH, Chklovskii DB. Wiring optimization can relate neuronal structure and function. Proceedings of the National Academy of Sciences of the United States of America. 2006;**103**(12):4723-4728. DOI: 10.1073/pnas.0506806103. Epub 2006 Mar 14

[37] Micheva KD, Smith SJ. Array tomography: A new tool for imaging the molecular architecture and ultrastructure of neural circuits. Neuron. 2007;**55**(1):25-36. DOI: 10.1016/j.neuron.2007.06.014

[38] Palm C, Axer M, Gräßel D, Dammers J, Lindemeyer J, Zilles K, et al. Towards ultra-high resolution fibre tract mapping of the human brain - registration of polarised light images and reorientation of fibre vectors. Frontiers in Human Neuroscience. 2010;**4**:9. DOI: 10.3389/neuro.09.009.2010

[39] Axer M, Amunts K, Grässel D, Palm C, Dammers J, Axer H, et al. A novel approach to the human connectome: Ultra-high resolution mapping of fiber tracts in the brain.

NeuroImage. 2011;**54**(2):1091-1101. DOI: 10.1016/j.neuroimage.2010.08.075. Epub 2010 Sep 9

[40] Fox MD, Raichle ME. Spontaneous fluctuations in brain activity observed with functional magnetic resonance imaging. Nature Reviews. Neuroscience. 2007;**8**(9):700-711. DOI: 10.1038/nrn2201

[41] Christova P, James LM, Georgopoulos AP. Effects of sex and age on presumed inhibitory interactions in 6 areas of the human cerebral cortex as revealed by the fMRI human connectome project. Experimental Brain Research. 2022;**240**(3):969-979. DOI: 10.1007/s00221-021-06298-z. Epub 2022 Jan 30

[42] Kim HG, Shin NY, Nam Y, Yun E, Yoon U, Lee HS, et al. MRI-visible dilated perivascular space in the brain by age: The human connectome project. Radiology. 2022;**213254**:1-9. DOI: 10.1148/radiol.213254. Epub ahead of print

[43] Chin Fatt CR, Jha MK, Minhajuddin A, Mayes T, Trivedi MH. Sex-specific differences in the association between body mass index and brain aging in young adults: Findings from the human connectome project. Psychoneuroendocrinology. 2021;**124**:105059. DOI: 10.1016/j.psyneuen.2020.105059. Epub 2020 Nov 16

[44] Wang Q, Akram H, Muthuraman M, Gonzalez-Escamilla G, Sheth SA, Oxenford S, et al. Normative vs. patient-specific brain connectivity in deep brain stimulation. Neuroimage. 2021;**224**:117307. DOI: 10.1016/j.neuroimage.2020.117307. Epub 2020 Aug 28

[45] Horn A, Reich M, Vorwerk J, Li N, Wenzel G, Fang Q, et al. Connectivity predicts deep brain stimulation outcome in Parkinson disease. Annals of Neurology. 2017;**82**(1):67-78. DOI: 10.1002/ana.24974

[46] Germann J, Elias GJB, Boutet A, Narang K, Neudorfer C, Horn A, et al. Brain structures and networks responsible for stimulation-induced memory flashbacks during forniceal deep brain stimulation for Alzheimer's disease. Alzheimer's & Dementia. 2021;**17**(5):777-787. DOI: 10.1002/alz.12238. Epub 2021 Jan 21

[47] Van Essen DC, Smith SM, Barch DM, Behrens TE, Yacoub E. Ugurbil K; WU-Minn HCP consortium. The WU-Minn human connectome project: An overview. NeuroImage. 2013;**80**:62-79. DOI: 10.1016/j.neuroimage.2013.05.041. Epub 2013 May 16

[48] Glasser MF, Smith SM, Marcus DS, Andersson JL, Auerbach EJ, Behrens TE, et al. The human connectome Project's neuroimaging approach. Nature Neuroscience. 2016;**19**(9):1175-1187. DOI: 10.1038/nn.4361

[49] Elam JS, Glasser MF, Harms MP, Sotiropoulos SN, Andersson JLR, Burgess GC, et al. The human connectome project: A retrospective. NeuroImage. 2021;**244**:118543. DOI: 10.1016/j.neuroimage.2021.118543. Epub 2021 Sep 8

[50] Merabet LB, Kobayashi M, Barton J, Pascual-Leone A. Suppression of complex visual hallucinatory experiences by occipital transcranial magnetic stimulation: A case report. Neurocase. 2003;**9**(5):436-440. DOI: 10.1076/neur.9.5.436.16557

[51] Henderson F, Abdullah KG, Verma R, Brem S. Tractography and the connectome in neurosurgical treatment of gliomas: The premise, the progress, and the potential. Neurosurgical Focus. 2020;**48**(2):E6. DOI: 10.3171/2019.11.FOCUS19785

[52] Chen Z, Ye N, Teng C, Li X. Alternations and applications of the

structural and functional connectome in gliomas: A mini-review. Frontiers in Neuroscience. 2022;**16**:856808. DOI: 10.3389/fnins.2022.856808

[53] Taylor PN, Sinha N, Wang Y, Vos SB, de Tisi J, Miserocchi A, et al. The impact of epilepsy surgery on the structural connectome and its relation to outcome. Neuroimage Clinical. 2018;**18**:202-214. DOI: 10.1016/j.nicl.2018.01.028

[54] Arski ON, Martire DJ, Young JM, Wong SM, Suresh H, Kerr EN, et al. Connectomic profiles and cognitive trajectories after epilepsy surgery in children. Neurology. 2022;**98**(22): e2233-e2244. DOI: 10.1212/WNL.0000000000200273. Epub 2022 Apr 11

[55] Chen X, Wang Y, Kopetzky SJ, Butz-Ostendorf M, Kaiser M. Connectivity within regions characterizes epilepsy duration and treatment outcome. Human Brain Mapping. 2021;**42**(12):3777-3791. DOI: 10.1002/hbm.25464. Epub 2021 May 11

[56] Englot DJ, Konrad PE, Morgan VL. Regional and global connectivity disturbances in focal epilepsy, related neurocognitive sequelae, and potential mechanistic underpinnings. Epilepsia. 2016;**57**(10):1546-1557. DOI: 10.1111/epi.13510. Epub 2016 Aug 24

[57] McIntyre CC, Savasta M, Kerkerian-Le Goff L, Vitek JL. Uncovering the mechanism(s) of action of deep brain stimulation: Activation, inhibition, or both. Clinical Neurophysiology. 2004;**115**(6):1239-1248. DOI: 10.1016/j.clinph.2003.12.024

[58] Lozano AM, Lipsman N, Bergman H, Brown P, Chabardes S, Chang JW, et al. Deep brain stimulation: Current challenges and future directions. Nature Reviews. Neurology. 2019;**15**(3):148-160. DOI: 10.1038/s41582-018-0128-2

[59] Horn A, Ostwald D, Reisert M, Blankenburg F. The structural-functional connectome and the default mode network of the human brain. NeuroImage. 2014;**102**(Pt 1):142-151. DOI: 10.1016/j.neuroimage.2013.09.069. Epub 2013 Oct 4

[60] Horn A, Kühn AA. Lead-DBS: A toolbox for deep brain stimulation electrode localizations and visualizations. NeuroImage. 2015;**107**:127-135. DOI: 10.1016/j.neuroimage.2014.12.002. Epub 2014 Dec 8

[61] Treu S, Strange B, Oxenford S, Neumann WJ, Kühn A, Li N, et al. Deep brain stimulation: Imaging on a group level. NeuroImage. 2020;**219**:117018. DOI: 10.1016/j.neuroimage.2020.117018. Epub 2020 Jun 4

[62] Mädler B, Coenen VA. Explaining clinical effects of deep brain stimulation through simplified target-specific modeling of the volume of activated tissue. AJNR. American Journal of Neuroradiology. 2012;**33**(6):1072-1080. DOI: 10.3174/ajnr.A2906. Epub 2012 Feb 2

[63] Dergachyova O, Zhao Y, Haegelen C, Jannin P, Essert C. Automatic preoperative planning of DBS electrode placement using anatomo-clinical atlases and volume of tissue activated. International Journal of Computer Assisted Radiology and Surgery. 2018;**13**(7):1117-1128. DOI: 10.1007/s11548-018-1724-8. Epub 2018 Mar 20

[64] Sobesky L, Goede L, Odekerken VJJ, Wang Q, Li N, Neudorfer C, et al. Subthalamic and pallidal deep brain stimulation: Are we modulating the same network? Brain. 2022;**145**(1):251-262. DOI: 10.1093/brain/awab258

[65] Kühn AA, Fogelson N, Limousin PD, Hariz MI, Kupsch A, Brown P. Frequency-specific effects of stimulation of the subthalamic area in treated Parkinson's disease patients. Neuroreport. 2009;**20**(11):975-978. DOI: 10.1097/WNR.0b013e32832d2456

[66] Kühn AA, Kempf F, Brücke C, Gaynor Doyle L, Martinez-Torres I, Pogosyan A, et al. High-frequency stimulation of the subthalamic nucleus suppresses oscillatory beta activity in patients with Parkinson's disease in parallel with improvement in motor performance. The Journal of Neuroscience. 2008;**28**(24):6165-6173. DOI: 10.1523/JNEUROSCI.0282-08.2008

[67] Tinkhauser G, Pogosyan A, Tan H, Herz DM, Kühn AA, Brown P. Beta burst dynamics in Parkinson's disease OFF and ON dopaminergic medication. Brain. 2017;**140**(11):2968-2981. DOI: 10.1093/brain/awx252

[68] Kühn AA, Tsui A, Aziz T, Ray N, Brücke C, Kupsch A, et al. Pathological synchronisation in the subthalamic nucleus of patients with Parkinson's disease relates to both bradykinesia and rigidity. Experimental Neurology. 2009;**215**(2):380-387. DOI: 10.1016/j.expneurol.2008.11.008. Epub 2008 Nov 25

[69] Kühn AA, Kupsch A, Schneider GH, Brown P. Reduction in subthalamic 8-35 Hz oscillatory activity correlates with clinical improvement in Parkinson's disease. The European Journal of Neuroscience. 2006;**23**(7):1956-1960. DOI: 10.1111/j.1460-9568.2006.04717.x

[70] Accolla EA, Herrojo Ruiz M, Horn A, Schneider GH, Schmitz-Hübsch T, Draganski B, et al. Brain networks modulated by subthalamic nucleus deep brain stimulation. Brain. 2016;**139** (Pt 9):2503-2515. DOI: 10.1093/brain/aww182. Epub 2016 Jul 13

[71] Hirschmann J, Özkurt TE, Butz M, Homburger M, Elben S, Hartmann CJ, et al. Differential modulation of STN-cortical and cortico-muscular coherence by movement and levodopa in Parkinson's disease. NeuroImage. 2013;**68**:203-213. DOI: 10.1016/j.neuroimage.2012.11.036. Epub 2012 Dec 16

[72] Tsuboi T, Charbel M, Peterside DT, Rana M, Elkouzi A, Deeb W, et al. Pallidal connectivity profiling of stimulation-induced dyskinesia in Parkinson's disease. Movement Disorders. 2021;**36**(2):380-388. DOI: 10.1002/mds.28324. Epub 2020 Oct 1

[73] Lofredi R, Auernig GC, Irmen F, Nieweler J, Neumann WJ, Horn A, et al. Subthalamic stimulation impairs stopping of ongoing movements. Brain. 2021;**144**(1):44-52. DOI: 10.1093/brain/awaa341

[74] de Almeida Marcelino AL, Horn A, Krause P, Kühn AA, Neumann WJ. Subthalamic neuromodulation improves short-term motor learning in Parkinson's disease. Brain. 2019;**142**(8):2198-2206. DOI: 10.1093/brain/awz152

[75] Avecillas-Chasin JM, Honey CR. Modulation of Nigrofugal and Pallidofugal pathways in deep brain stimulation for Parkinson disease. Neurosurgery. 2020;**86**(4):E387-E397. DOI: 10.1093/neuros/nyz544

[76] Lizarraga KJ, Naghibzadeh M, Boutet A, Elias GJB, Fasano A. Management of Pisa syndrome with lateralized subthalamic stimulation. Journal of Neurology. 2018;**265**(10):2442-2444. DOI: 10.1007/s00415-018-8991-8. Epub 2018 Aug 3

[77] Irmen F, Horn A, Mosley P, Perry A, Petry-Schmelzer JN, Dafsari HS, et al. Left prefrontal connectivity links subthalamic stimulation with depressive

symptoms. Annals of Neurology. 2020;**87**(6):962-975. DOI: 10.1002/ana.25734. Epub 2020 Apr 30

[78] Cury RG, Teixeira MJ, Galhardoni R, Silva V, Iglesio R, França C, et al. Connectivity patterns of subthalamic stimulation influence pain outcomes in Parkinson's disease. Frontiers in Neurology. 2020;**11**:9. DOI: 10.3389/fneur.2020.00009

[79] Mosley PE, Paliwal S, Robinson K, Coyne T, Silburn P, Tittgemeyer M, et al. The structural connectivity of subthalamic deep brain stimulation correlates with impulsivity in Parkinson's disease. Brain. 2020;**143**(7):2235-2254. DOI: 10.1093/brain/awaa148

Chapter 4

# Stereotactic Electroencephalography (SEEG)

*See Ka Wing Michael*

## Abstract

Drug resistant epilepsy (DRE) is not an uncommon clinical condition. DRE could cause disabling seizures and even sudden unexpected death in epilepsy (SUDEP). Pre-surgical evaluation is necessary to for surgical treatment to cure or palliative epilepsy. If feasible, surgical excision of an epileptic focus provides the best chance of cure. However, the standard non-invasive workup could not always identify the epileptic focus. Stereotactic EEG (SEEG) is an invasive EEG that could provide the spatial and temporal progression of epileptic discharge so that we could localize or lateralise the epileptic focus more easily. This chapter aims to illustrate the principle of SEEG, the methods of SEEG electrode insertion, the usual white matter tract pathway that epileptic discharge progresses. It also discusses the therapeutic use of SEEG in lesioning with radiofrequency ablation (RFA), as well as the future potential as part of the brain-computer interface (BCI).

**Keywords:** stereotactic electroencephalography, drug-resistant epilepsy, radiofrequency ablation, neuroprosthesis, brain-computer interface

## 1. Introduction

Stereotactic electroencephalography (SEEG) is the study of the electrical activities of the brain by means of implantation of electrodes into brain parenchyma with the aid of stereotactic navigation [1].

It was first developed by Jean Talairach and Jean Bancaud in France in the late 1950s. Talairach was a renowned stereotactic neurosurgeon who developed the frame-based coordinate system of the human brain based on the anatomical AC-PC (anterior commissure – posterior commissure) line, while Bancaud put forth the presurgical evaluation of drug-resistant epilepsy (DRE) with the use of the Talariach method. Bancaud described the organization of temporal lobe seizure with respect to the mesial temporal structures and the temporal neocortex [2]. This laid the foundation of SEEG as the presurgical workup for refractory epilepsy. It was then used in France, Italy and Canada for some time.

Only till 2010s, it was adopted in the United States and gained popularity because of its attractive safety profile and the capacity to perform spatiotemporal analysis of the progression of the epileptiform discharge and bilateral cerebral hemisphere simultaneously, in comparison with subdural grid and depth electrodes which study cases that were already lateralized and/or partially localized [3].

Moreover, as the technology improves, SEEG could combine with lesioning technique to eradicate the epileptogenic zone, for example, radiofrequency ablation (RFA) [4]. This therapeutic use became more popular since the 2000s. Besides, as the electrodes were getting smaller and smaller, it had its potential in the application in brain-computer interface and the development of neuroprosthesis, in contrast to the traditional use of electrocorticography (ECoG).

Thus, this chapter aims to review the roles of SEEG as:

1. Diagnostic purpose in presurgical workup for drug-resistant epilepsy

2. Therapeutic use to lesion the epileptogenic zone

3. Potential use in brain-computer interface, to create neuroprosthesis

## 2. Diagnostic use

### 2.1 Definition and epileptogenesis

To start with, it is important to clarify the concepts of drug-resistant epilepsy (DRE), zonification of epileptogenesis, and a proper presurgical workup.

Drug-resistant epilepsy, aka medical refractory epilepsy, is defined as the failure of adequate trials of two well-tolerated, appropriately chosen and used antiepileptic drug schedules, be it monotherapy or polytherapy, according to the International League Against Epilepsy (ILAE) consensus in 2009 [5]. Patients with DRE is eligible for presurgical evaluation.

In case of focal epilepsy, an *epileptogenic zone* (EZ) may be identified where cure of epilepsy could be achieved if it is resected. For the terminology in epileptogenesis, *epileptogenic lesion* is the anatomical abnormality which could be identified in structural imaging such as MRI [6]. *Ictal onset zone* is the origin of the seizure which could be the brain parenchyma without the lesion. Epileptogenic lesion and the ictal onset zone, together, form the EZ. However, sometimes when the epileptiform discharges propagate to the other parts of the brain causing symptoms. Those part would be named *symptomatogenic zone*. Most of the time, the symptoms could be the more obvious part of the seizure semiology which could make the localization of the EZ confusing. For example, a temporal EZ could transmit the epileptiform discharge to the frontal lobe via white matter tracts such as uncinate fasciculus and arcuate fasciculus, leading to the clinical impression of frontal epilepsy. On the other hand, *irritative zone* refers to the area which produces interictal epileptiform discharge. *Functional deficit zone* refers to the area of hypometabolism in functional imaging i.e. interictal PET scan. Irritative and functional deficit zones could overlap with the EZ but the areas represented are often exaggerated. This zonification concept forms the foundation of *localization* of the culprit of the epilepsy (**Table 1**) (**Figure 1**). On the other hand, *lateralization* of the epilepsy to either left or right side is also crucial but could be difficult at times, especially in frontal epilepsy in which synchronization of the bilateral cerebral hemisphere could be quick via commissural fibers such as corpus callosum.

| | |
|---|---|
| Epileptogenic lesion | Anatomical abnormality in neuroimaging |
| Ictal onset zone | Onset of seizure |
| Epileptogenic zone | Epileptogenic lesion + Ictal onset zone |
| Symptomatogenic zone | Area which produces symptoms |
| Irritative zone | Area which produces interictal epileptiform discharge |
| Functional deficit zone | Area of hypometabolism in interictal functional imaging |

**Table 1.**
*Zonification of epileptogenesis.*

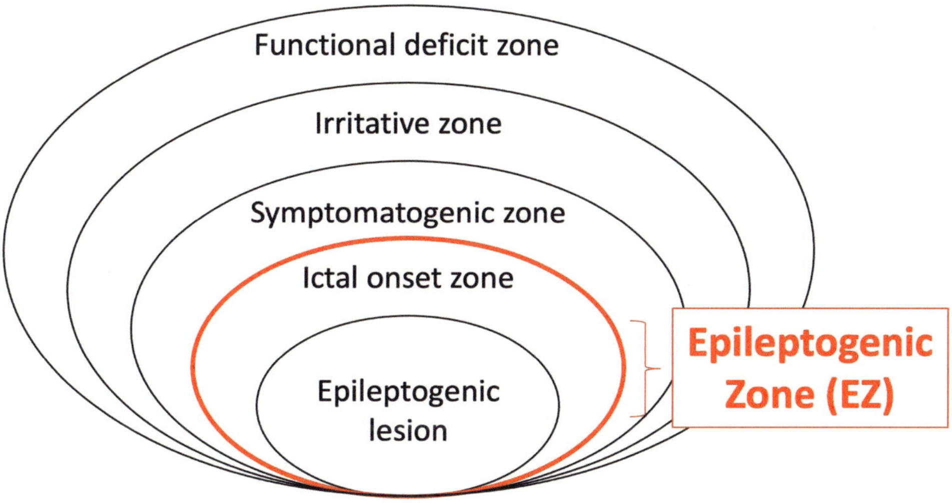


**Figure 1.**
*Zonification of epileptogenesis.*

## 2.2 Presurgical workup

A presurgical workup aims to generate an *anatomical-clinical-electrophysiological (ACE) hypothesis*. MRI, video EEG and neuropsychiatric assessment form the core of it. An MRI with good resolution would offer the *localization* of the epileptogenic lesion, which lays the foundation of good surgical outcome to start with, as lesional epilepsy has a better outcome (by two to three times) than non-lesional epilepsy after neurosurgical intervention [7]. 3-T MRI, which has a higher signal-to-noise ratio, could be more accurate in delineating the lesion as compare with 1.5-T MRI as illustrated in some qualitative studies [8]. An ictal video EEG would be more valuable than an interictal EEG because it offers the appreciation of the clinical semiology with the ictal discharges simultaneously, while interictal EEG could only illustrate the irritative zone. Neuropsychiatric assessment could offer evidence of brain dysfunction secondary to epileptic encephalopathy. For example, frontal lobe epilepsy might cause frontal lobe syndrome such as disinhibition, perseverance, etc. For temporal lobe epilepsy in dominant hemisphere, it causes more verbal memory deficit as compared with the visual memory deficit in the non-dominant hemisphere. It is often how *lateralization* is done in cases such as mesial temporal sclerosis. Bilateral mesial temporal sclerosis is not uncommon.

If these three investigations provide concordant findings, in which an EZ could be concluded, then surgical excision might be proceeded. The most often encountered example would be temporal lobe epilepsy secondary to mesial temporal sclerosis. Indeed, mesial temporal resection (i.e. amygdalohippocampectomy), via either transtemporal (anterior temporal lobectomy) or transsylvian approach, offer some of the best outcome in terms of seizure control.

Functional images such as interictal PET-CT could provide supportive information but often it is not conclusive due to its lack of spatial resolution. Nowadays, a PET-MRI could be done in the same setting to provide the simultaneous appreciation of anatomical and functional data, which might be more superior than fusing, by software, the interictal PET-CT with the MRI which were done in two settings. Ictal SPECT is also valuable to evaluate the part of brain with the greatest perfusion which is often the EZ. It is the most useful when there is more than one lesion, and the clinician could not conclude which one is the culprit. However, it is technically demanding as the radioactive isotope should be injected once the ictal event starts, in terms of seconds. Also, if the electrophysiological onset precedes the clinical one, the ictal event has started for some time before clinical semiology happens. For lateralization of dominant hemisphere, functional MRI by means of blood oxygen level dependent (BOLD) might be helpful to lateralize the language area. Yet, there could be bilateral activation at times especially in those who were agitated or intellectually disabled. Of note, even functional MRI could lateralize the language area, it has relatively poor spatial resolution as it is all about the adjustment of the threshold in the software. It could not replace the language assessment in awake craniotomy in case of proximity of the EZ to the language areas. Magnetoencephalography (MEG) is to detect dipoles which occur in the EZ. It is similar to SPECT but it is not as time-dependent.

If the above measures (some refer them as level 1) provide discordant findings (**Table 2**), and *lateralization* and *localization* could not be achieved, invasive workup (i.e. level 2) might have to be considered [9]. Wada test involves the endovascular injection of barbiturate to internal carotid artery (ICA) to temporarily suppress the activity of one cerebral hemisphere to see if it causes verbal or visual memory deficits, as mentioned, which then points to left or right-side temporal lobe epilepsy respectively. If ICA Wada test fails to lateralize the dominant hemisphere, then selective posterior cerebral artery (PCA) Wada test could be considered to selectively suppress the activity of the hippocampus [10].

### 2.3 Invasive EEG

Here comes to the invasive EEG. If an epilepsy is lateralized and partially localized in the level 1 presurgical workup, craniotomy for putting in subdural grid or depth electrodes (SDE) was the commonest method for invasive EEG. Subdural grid offers

| | |
|---|---|
| MRI | to localize the *epileptogenic lesion* |
| Ictal Video EEG | to localize the *ictal onset zone* and characterize the semiology which helps to localize the *symptomatogenic zone* |
| Interictal EEG | to localize the *irritative zone* |
| Neuropsychiatric assessment | to lateralize the epilepsy |
| Interictal PET | to localize the *functional deficit zone* |
| Ictal SPECT and MEG | to localize the *epileptogenic zone* |

**Table 2.**
*Level 1 presurgical workup.*

examination of epileptiform discharges across the cerebral convexity while depth electrodes provide the assessment of epileptiform discharges from deep to superficial. Yet, it involves the risks of bleeding and infection, especially in those with prior craniotomy. It might also cause unhabitual seizure events during the recording which might confuse the clinical picture.

Stereotactic EEG (SEEG) involves the minimally invasive approach to implant multiple electrodes with twist drill to cover different areas of a cerebral hemisphere. Bilateral implantation is also feasible. Simultaneous deep and superficial assessment of multiple sites is one of its greatest advantages [11]. The spatial and temporal relationship of the epileptiform discharges as in a 3D coordinate system could be delineated. The epileptic network could be determined. It causes less unhabitual seizure event. In the series by McGonigal A, *et al.*, SEEG localizes the EZ in non-lesional epilepsy cases as effective as in lesional ones [12]. In the meta-analysis published by Mullin, *et al.*, the bleeding and infection rate was found to be 1% and 0.8% respectively [13]. In the meta-analysis by Arya R. *et al.*, the rate was 4% and 2.3% respectively [14]. In some lesional cases with anatomical discordance (e.g., right temporal lobe epilepsy with a deeper pathology hypothalamic hamartoma), or when there are multiple pathologies (e.g., polymicrogyria, periventricular nodular heterotopia), SEEG could be helpful to identify or confirm the true pathology that is responsible for the epileptogenesis [15]. At the moment, there is no head-to-head series to compare the seizure control rate between SEEG and SDE. According to the review by Katz JS *et al.*, there is no definite superiority of SEEG vs. SDE (Engel class I rate 56–68% vs. 30–70%) with reference to different case series [16].

There are three ways to implant SEEG, namely frameless, frame-based and robotic-assisted stereotactic navigation. Frameless navigation system makes use of guidance by neuroimaging with surface matching registration. Frame-based approach involves the application of stereotactic frame to patient's head. Fusion of post-frame CT scan with the initial planning MRI will provide the coordinates with reference to the stereotactic frame to navigate the intended trajectory. Robotic-assisted stereotactic navigation also involves registration but it differs by having robot to bring neurosurgeons to the intended trajectory, which could speed up the procedure when there are multiple electrodes to be inserted, as in the case of SEEG. In the meta-analysis performed by Vejay N. Vakharia *et al.* in 2017, the mean error of the entry point and target point was 2.45 and 2.89 mm for frameless approach, 1.43 and 1.93 mm for frame-based approach, and 1.17 and 1.71 mm for robotic-assisted approach [17]. Despite the apparently smaller mean error in frame-based and robotic-assisted approaches, there was high heterogeneity among studies and the parameters used were different (Euclidean distance vs. lateral deviation). This precluded meaningful comparison of the different approaches.

### 2.4 SEEG planning

The flow of the SEEG planning and implantation procedures is as follows. At the combined epilepsy meeting, the findings of the presurgical workup are presented and the plan for SEEG is confirmed in selected cases with discordant findings. Multidisciplinary discussion to generate the anatomical-clinical-electrophysiological hypothesis would be essential. Implantation of electrodes would depend on the best hypothesis generated and important alternative hypothesis to be rejected. A 2D grid coordinate system (aka Talairach Stereotactic System) might be helpful for communication among the team (**Figure 2**). Fine-cut MRI brain with contrast would be

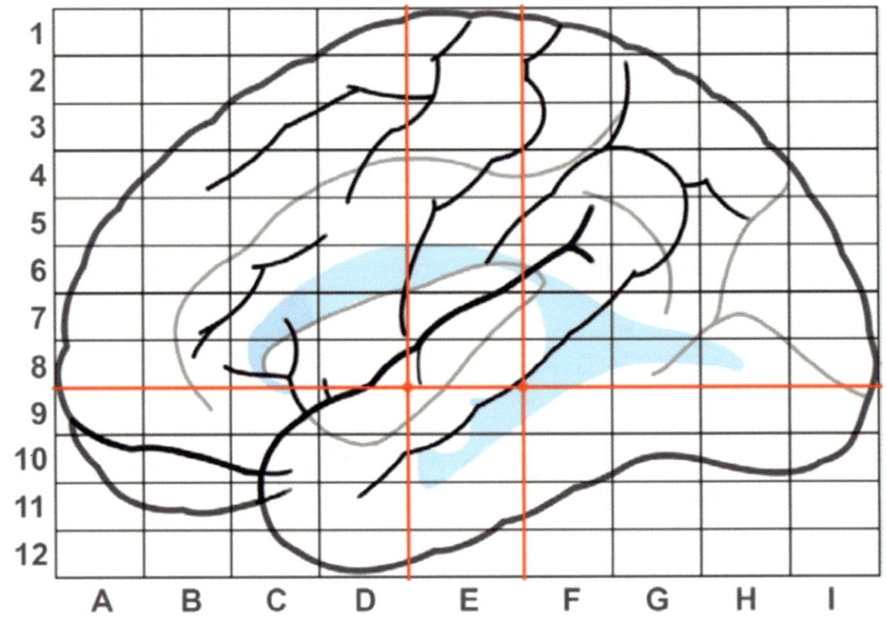


**Figure 2.**
*Talairach stereotactic system.*

used for stereotactic navigation and trajectory planning. A CT cerebral angiogram would be useful to appreciate the bony architecture as well as the cortical and Sylvian vessels. MRI with cerebral angiogram (MRA) fusing with a plain CT brain is also an alternative to reduce contrast use.

In the planning software, we could put the trajectories in an orthogonal manner i.e., perpendicular to mid-sagittal plane of the brain. It is similar to the Talairach approach, yet the latter made use of 2D angiography (digital subtraction angiography). The patient would be positioned laterally during the implantation procedure. Orthogonal approach has the advantage of easier interpretation of the spread of the epileptiform discharges as the 3D system could be more regular in shape if all the electrodes are parallel to each other. However, the more peripheral the SEEG electrodes are, there could be greater deviation as the electrode direction is not perpendicular to the skull and the brain surface which could lead to deviation towards the periphery. Therefore, the region of interest of the procedure must be determined and marked during the planning and the setup of the navigation system. Of course, the region of interest is often the proposed EZ. On the other hand, orthogonal insertion to insula could be difficult. Insula is often the important alternative to exclude in both frontal and temporal epilepsy. Anatomically it is covered by frontal, temporal, and parietal operculum with Sylvian fissure and middle cerebral artery (MCA) branches on the surface. Therefore, the orthogonal insertion to insula region needs great care not to pass through important vasculature. However, it allows the simultaneous assessment of both operculum and the insula on the same electrode. The other way to implant the SEEG would be a 3D approach, adjusting to the skull shape at the entry site (**Figures 3** and **4**) and to avoid MCA branches in Sylvian fissure in case the insula is one of the targets (**Figure 5**). Yet, as the electrodes are not parallel to each other, interpretation could be more difficult.

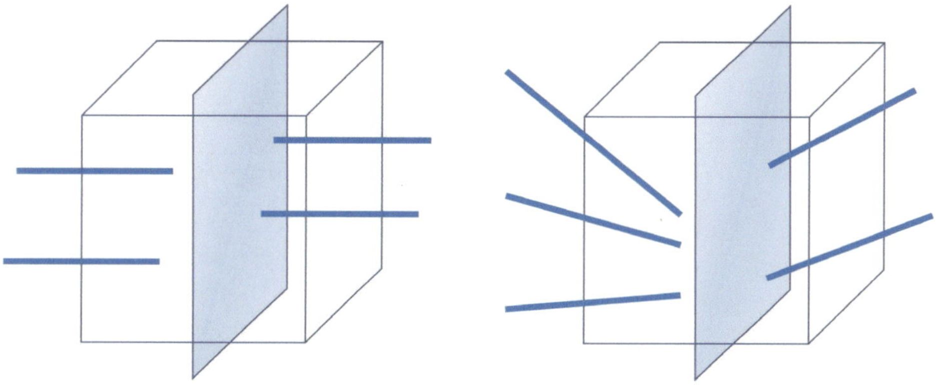

**Figure 3.**
*Comparison of orthogonal (left) with 3D (right) approach.*

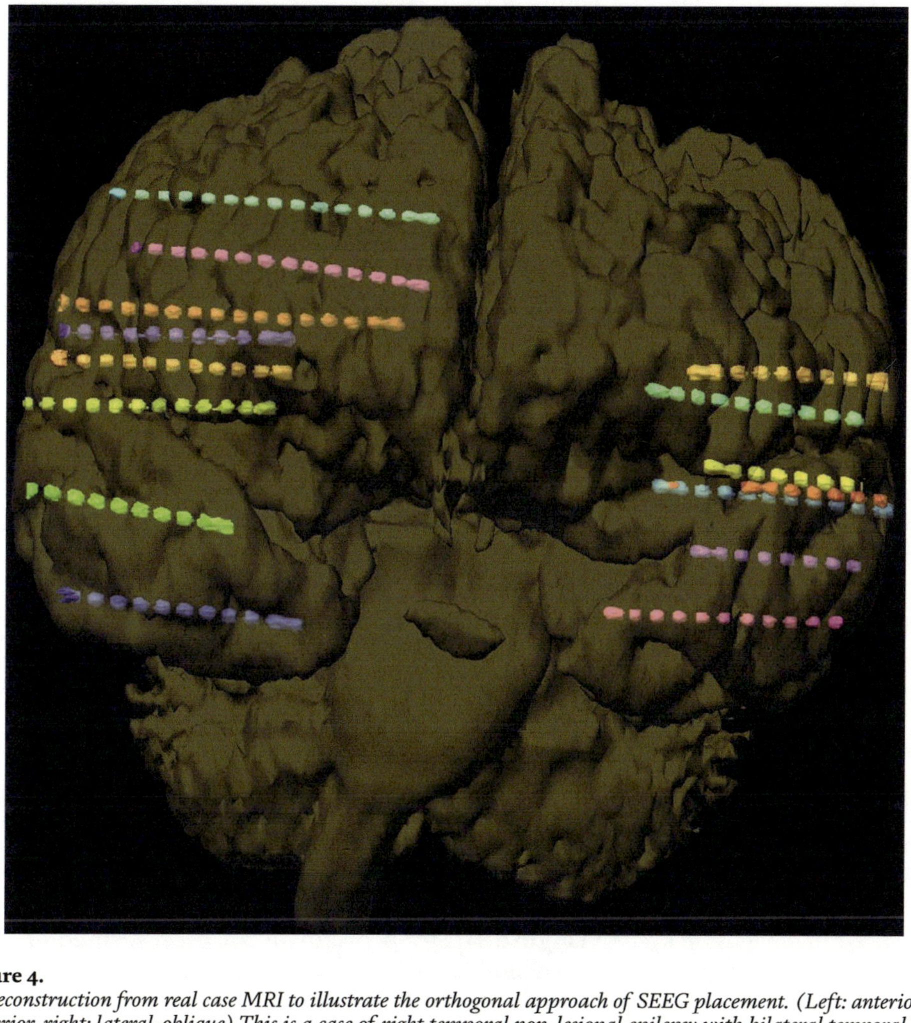

**Figure 4.**
*3D reconstruction from real case MRI to illustrate the orthogonal approach of SEEG placement. (Left: anterior-posterior, right: lateral-oblique) This is a case of right temporal non-lesional epilepsy with bilateral temporal EEG onset and MEG dipoles with semiology of cephalic aura, bilateral hearing loss followed by left side twitching.*

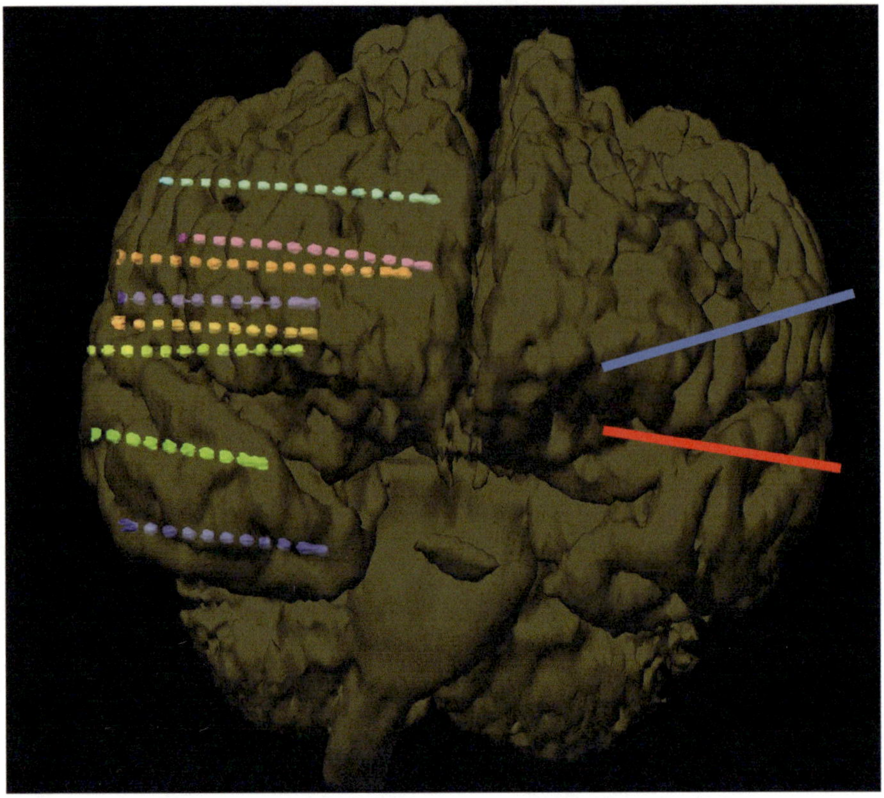

**Figure 5.**
*This is an anterior-posterior view of the 3D-reconstructed brain parenchyma. Blue line represents the 3D approach which avoids the Sylvian fissure while the red line represents the orthogonal approach which punctures through the Sylvian fissure.*

The planning strategy in different epilepsy would be discussed in later part. During the planning, entry sites and target sites must be determined. Then the length from dura to target should be measured. Many of the planning software could customize the lead contact size and intervals. With reference to the insert of the electrodes, one could decide the length of different electrodes to be used. After planning the trajectories in the planning software, either frameless stereotactic navigation system or robotic-assisted system could be used directly. Frame-based approach would require a post-frame CT.

## 2.5 SEEG implantation

Patient is then put under general anesthesia and intubation. Head is secured by clamp and navigation system is set. Skin is prepared and draped. Adjustment of the guiding system is performed (**Figure 6**). The length inserted would be calculated with reference to the different parts of the system (**Figure 7**). Skin-dura distance is measured in navigation system (**Figure 8**). Stopper-skin distance is measured intra-operatively. Adding the two up we would have the length of drill needed to puncture the skull. Stab wound is made on the scalp. Drill with length marked by stopper is brought in. Skull is drilled (**Figure 9**). Sometimes 1–2 mm more might be needed to puncture the inner table. A sense of give-way under careful control is often the sign

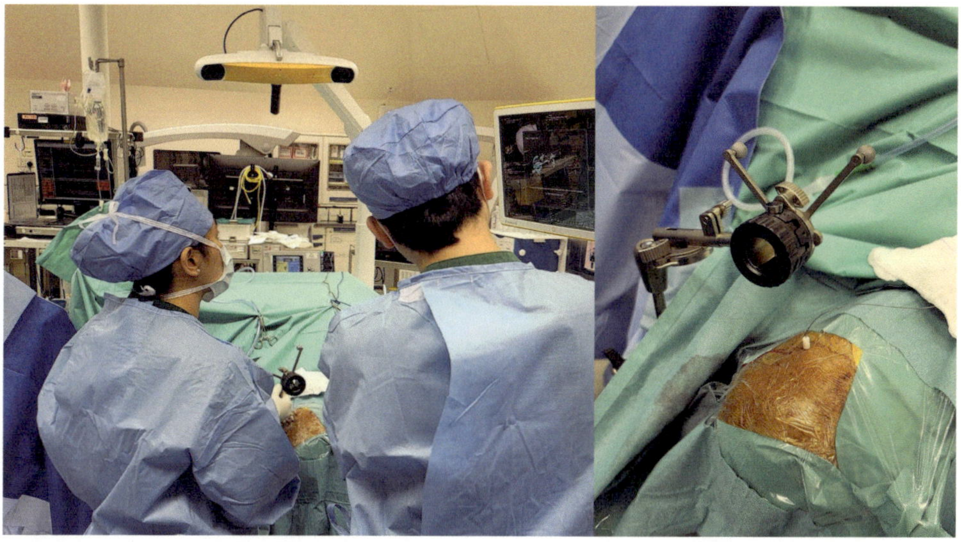

**Figure 6.**
*Guiding system is adjusted by frameless stereotactic navigation.*

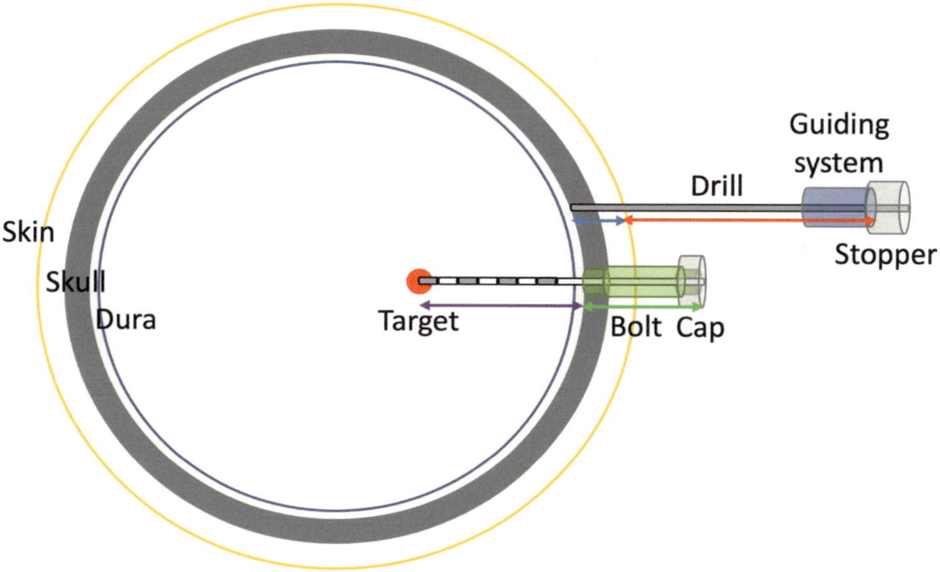


**Figure 7.**
*Blue arrows = skin-dura distance. Red arrows = stopper to skin distance. Blue + red = length of drill to puncture the skull. Purple arrows = dura-target distance. Green arrows = bolt-dura distance. Purple + green = length of electrode.*

of complete puncture. Dura and pia are cauterized and punctured by monopolar (**Figure 10**). The bolt is anchored to the skull. Length of electrode is needed is the sum of dura-target distance and the bolt-dura distance (i.e., from bolt to target). The electrode with length marked by the cap is inserted with the cap screwed to the bolt (**Figure 11**). Opposition of the scalp wounds might be needed to prevent CSF leak. The whole procedure is repeated in different electrodes. In case of bilateral

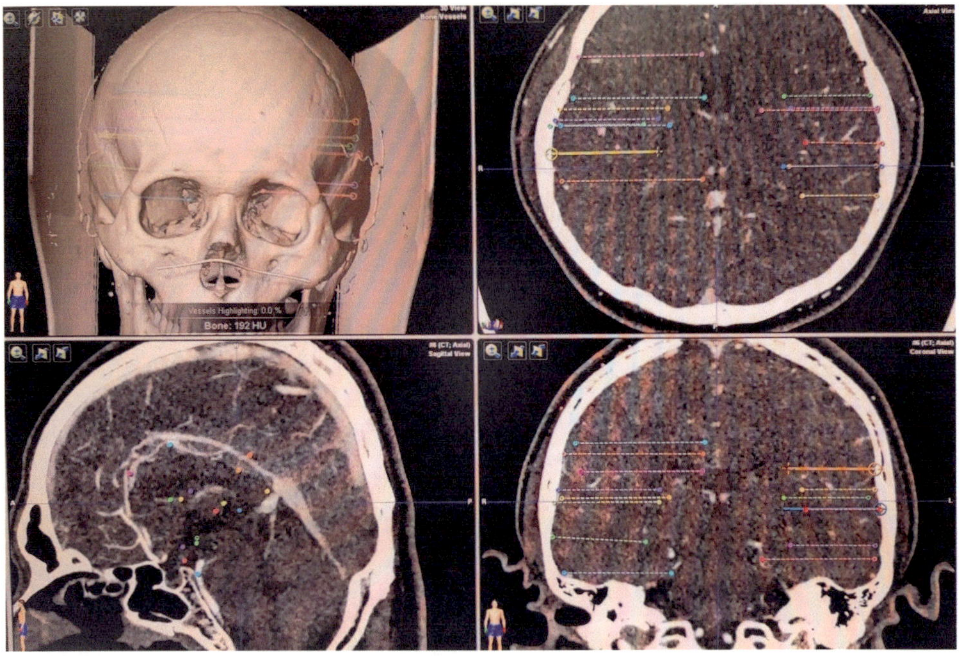


**Figure 8.**
*Electrodes are planned in orthogonal manner. Skin-dura distance could be measured.*

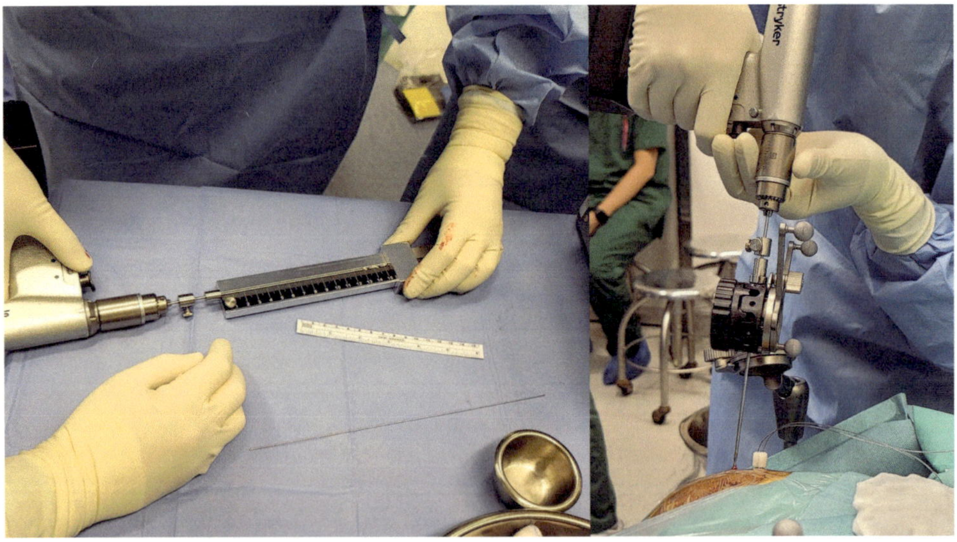


**Figure 9.**
*Stopper-dura distance is set. Bone drilling.*

implantation, the patient would be repositioned in the contralateral side, in lateral position, with navigation system set again. It should be reminded that the EEG signals recorded intraoperatively might be affected by the general anesthesia. Patient would be transferred back to the ward for monitoring of the SEEG signals (**Figure 12**). In author's center, we put patients on empirical antibiotics when the patient is under the

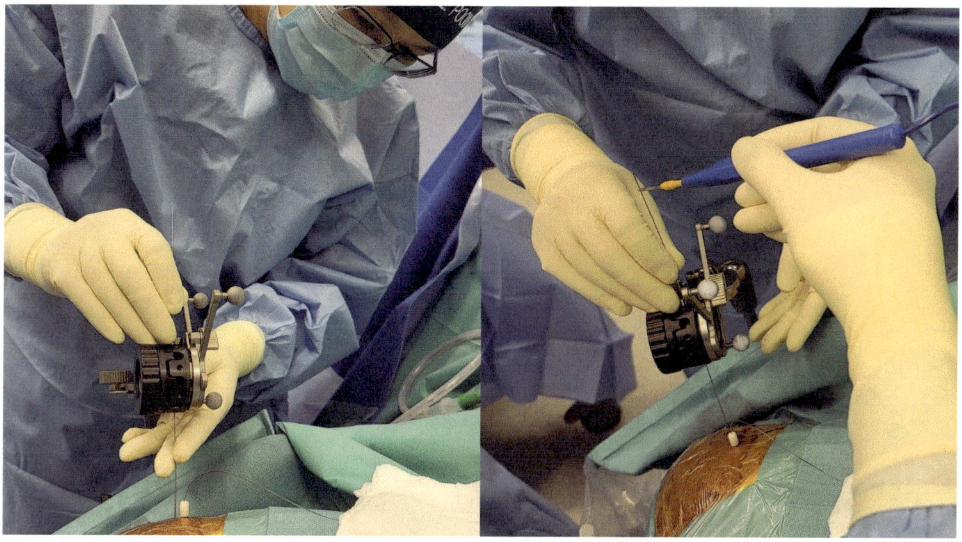

**Figure 10.**
*Dura cauterization and puncture.*

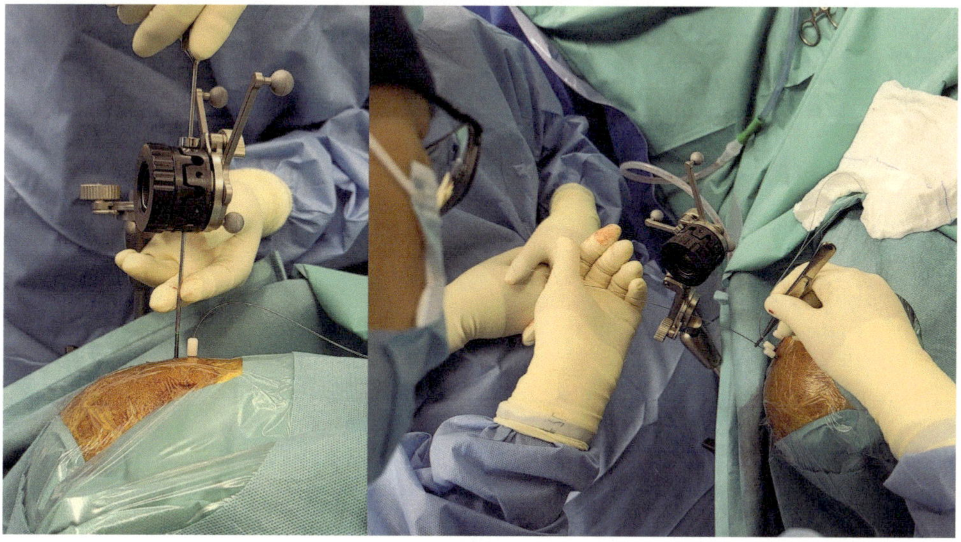

**Figure 11.**
*Bolt anchoring and electrode insertion.*

SEEG monitoring. Antiepileptics would be withheld according to the patient's semiology and seizure frequency. CSF leak is what one should carefully watch out for.

### 2.6 SEEG signal recording and stimulation

Post-operative CT scan would be fused to the preoperative MRI. First, we assess the accuracy of electrodes placement. Second, the electrodes are segmented, and the anatomical position of different contacts are marked. SEEG signals would be recorded by 4–5 days. By then stimulation might be performed. On one hand seizure events

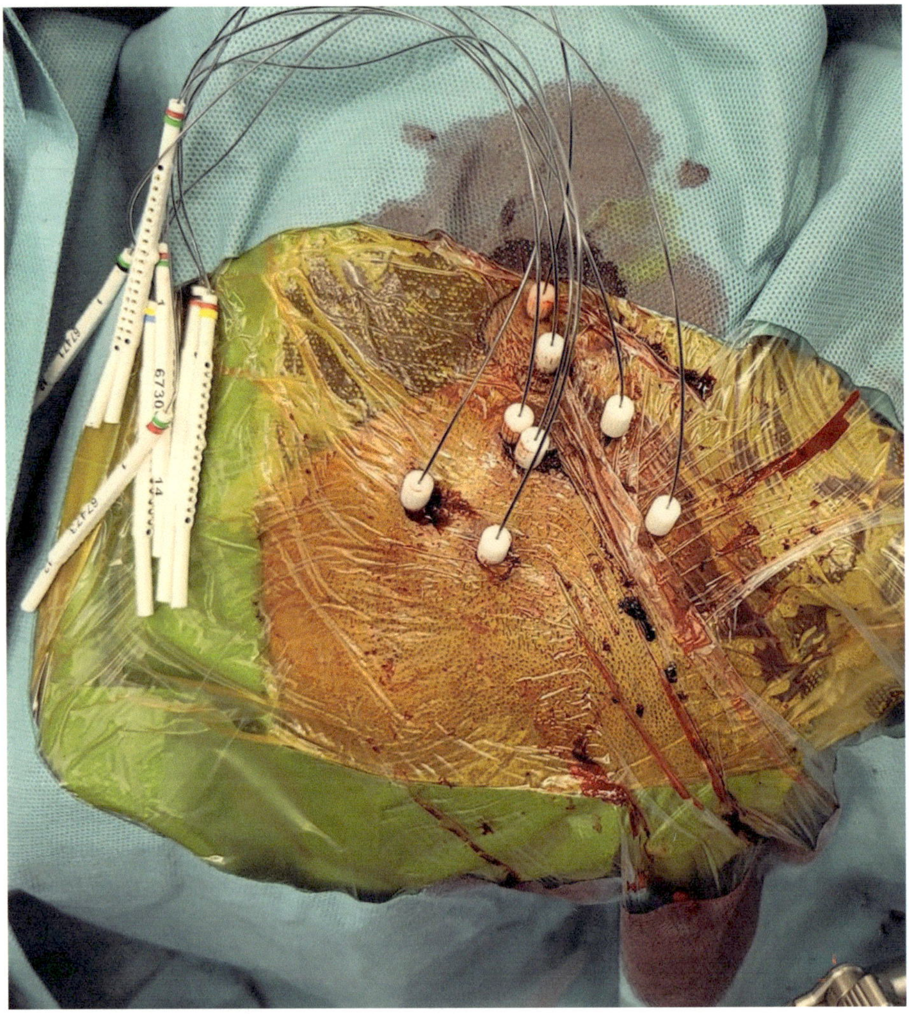

**Figure 12.**
*Electrodes are ready for connection to EEG montage. Betadine-soaked dressing is applied.*

could be triggered to give clinicians a hint on the location of the ictal onset zone. Yet, the events might be unhabitual. On the other hand, some eloquent areas might be located by the stimulation. Concerning the stimulation technique, low frequency stimulation (1 Hz frequency, 0.5-4 mA pulse intensity, 0.5-3 ms pulse width, 20–60s duration) is suitable for areas of low after-discharge threshold such as primary auditory cortex, primary motor cortex, hippocampus, and areas with focal cortical dysplasia. High frequency stimulation (50 Hz, 0.5-5 mA, 0.5-1 ms, 3–8 s) would be suitable to areas elsewhere [18]. Stimulation might be helpful for clinicians to understand the epileptic network better (**Figure 13**).

## 2.7 Removal of leads and resection epilepsy surgery

Once the anatomical-clinical-electrophysiological hypothesis is made after the discussion in the multidisciplinary team, one could proceed to removal of the SEEG

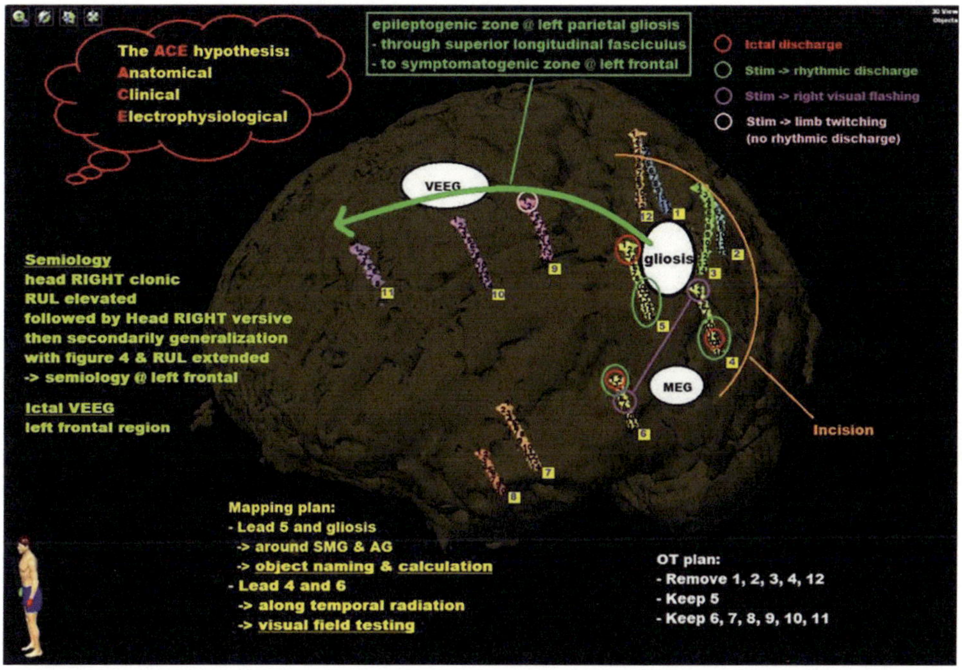


**Figure 13.**
*This diagram illustrates a case with epileptogenic zone confirmed with direct electrical stimulation. The epileptogenic lesion was the gliosis with T2 hyperintensity in MRI in the temporoparietal junction. Yet, the patient's semiology was often a frontal one. SEEG electrodes were implanted around the gliosis and the dipoles found in MEG. They were also implanted across the superior longitudinal fasciculus. Stimulation triggers rhythmic discharge in the superficial contacts around the gliosis and thus identifies the ictal onset zone. Visual pathway was also identified in the deeper contacts of one adjacent electrode.*

leads and excision of the EZ. Usually, the leads inserted to the proposed EZ would be removed first to provide the surgical exposure. The remaining leads could be left to detect any interictal signals. If they are present, they could serve as a guide to successful disconnection of the EZ once they disappeared. However, one should not compromise the surgical exposure which is critical to adequate excision of the EZ and careful hemostasis. Awake craniotomy might be needed for assessment of the eloquent areas with direct electrical stimulation to avoid neurological deficits after the operation. Awake craniotomy might even need a larger exposure for adequate assessment. Details of awake craniotomy would be out of the scope of this chapter. As the leads have been implanted for 1–2 weeks before the concluding procedure, risk of infection could be higher than usual craniotomy cases. Therefore, intra-operative wound irrigation and post-operative antibiotics might also be helpful.

## 2.8 Implantation strategy

SEEG electrodes should be implanted according to the anatomical-clinical-electro-physiological hypothesis [19]. It is also important to place electrodes, apart from the proposed EZ, the symptomatogenic and functional deficit zones.

Temporal lobe epilepsy (TLE), as mentioned, with mesial temporal sclerosis and concordant presurgical workup, could have resection surgery proceeded right away. However, the following four situations might warrant SEEG implantation.

1. Presurgical workup is discordant (e.g. a left TLE semiology with right mesial temporal sclerosis)

2. TLE is bilateral.

3. TLE with extratemporal epileptic generator e.g.

    a. Orbitofrontal structures (spread via uncinate fasciculus)

    b. Posterior cortices i.e. parietal and occipital (spread via inferior frontal-occipital fasciculus or inferior longitudinal fasciculus)

4. TLE-plus with early involving of neighboring structures

    a. Orbitofrontal structures

    b. Insular cortex, frontal operculum

    c. Temporo-parieto-occipital junction

From these one could appreciate in TLE, orbitofrontal structures and insula are two very important structures to have the electrodes stationed. Understanding the connectome with the white matter tracts is also essential as it is often how epileptiform discharges spread (**Figure 14**).

For frontal lobe epilepsy, the epileptiform discharges often spread quickly within the frontal lobe, and it has high connectivity with the extra-frontal structures and the contralateral frontal lobe. SEEG is mainly to compartmentalize the seizure pattern. The frontal operculum could be divided into the pars orbitalis, pars triangularis and opercularis. Orthogonal insertion of the SEEG electrode into the pars orbitalis could provide assessment of the orbitofrontal structures. On the other hand, mesial frontal structures are often underrepresented in scalp EEG. Orthogonal insertion of the SEEG electrodes via middle frontal gyrus often provide assessment of that with the deeper contacts. Therefore, if frontal lobe is of concern and mesial frontal structures must be assessed, a longer electrode might have to be used.

Posterior quadrant epilepsy is a less frequently encountered type. It involves parietal and occipital lobes. Clinical polymorphism is present due to high density of brain connections to the insula and temporal as well as contralateral posterior quadrant. It is often some challenging cases and multi-lobar and bilateral electrodes might have to be used to assess the propagation pathways and assessment of the functional areas such as Wernicke's area, reading, calculation, vision, and face recognition. Tractography study such as diffusion tensor imaging (DTI) might be helpful to look for the ventral and dorsal white matter tracts through the occipital lobe. SEEG electrodes could be implanted according to the white matter tracts and see if the epileptiform discharge propagates from one to another electrode via the pathway.

Insular epilepsy has the semiology mimicking frontal and temporal lobe epilepsy. As mentioned, it is often an important alterative to exclude. Again, it is underrepresented in scalp electrodes. Difficulty to plan trajectories of the SEEG electrodes is often encountered due to the vascular constraints, especially with the orthogonal approach. The comparison of orthogonal and 3D approaches is discussed in previous part.

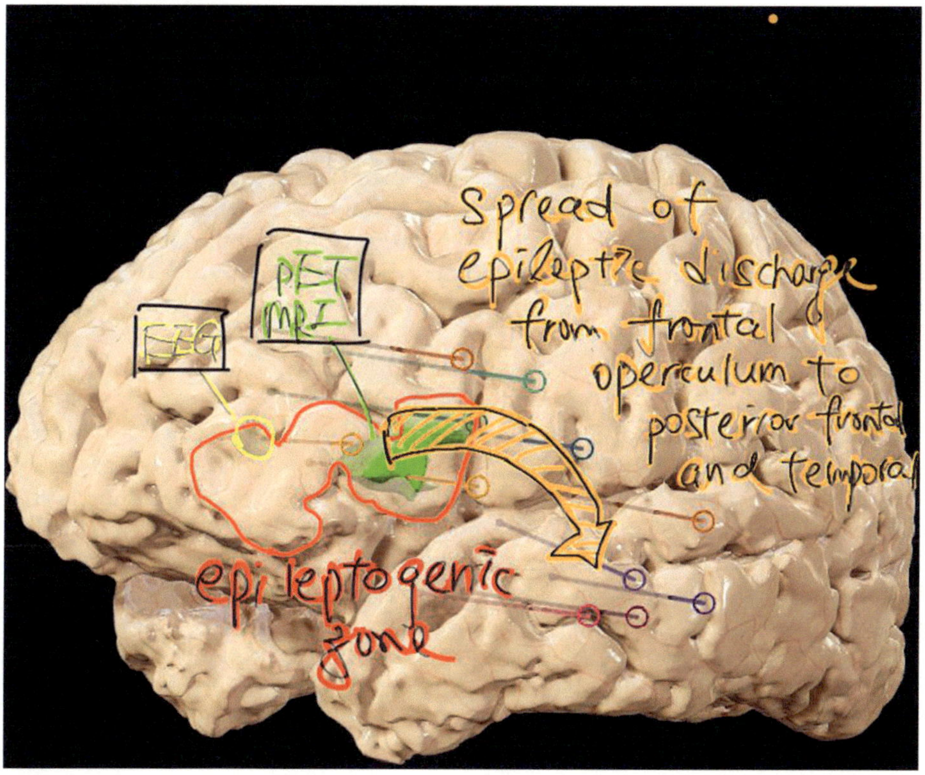


**Figure 14.**
*An illustration of a case of temporal lobe epilepsy semiology with hand and oral automatism followed by post-ictal drowsiness yet EZ concluded to be in the orbitofrontal structures with spread to temporal lobe via pathways such as uncinate fasciculus or arcuate fasciculus. SEEG concluded the ictal onset zone (yellow) while the PET-MRI confirmed the functional deficit zone (green). Electrodes were also inserted in an orthogonal approach to the insula as it is an important alternative hypothesis to exclude.*

## 3. Therapeutic use

### 3.1 Radiofrequency ablation (RFA)

Stereotactic lesioning has long been a surgical treatment to focal epilepsy. Examples include laser interstitial thermal therapy (LITT) and SEEG-coupled RFA. Lesioning technique is more suitable for lesional epilepsy as the lesion could be identified and approached by the SEEG electrode, whereas in non-lesional epilepsy, the electrodes are often placed according to the epileptogenic network. It could be helpful in cases when open surgery is relatively contraindicated. For example, in temporal lobe epilepsy in dominant hemisphere, stereotactic lesioning might be able to treat the mesial temporal structure where a dominant hippocampectomy is contraindicated. On the other hand, deeply located pathology such as hypothalamic hamartoma and periventricular nodular heterotopia could be treated by stereotaxic lesioning instead of making large corticotomy or passing through important structures such as basal ganglia. More importantly, stereotactic lesioning is *not* a contraindication to subsequent surgery i.e., resection or neuromodulation. SEEG-guided RFA is done by applying radiofrequency thermocoagulation between two contiguous electrode contacts to make a precise lesion. SEEG signals would be recorded and the likely ictal onset zone together with the MRI-found epileptogenic lesion would be concluded to be the EZ. Direct electric stimulation as previously discussed could also give us the guidance of where the EZ is and if any eloquent areas are nearby. When the target of lesioning is decided, power would be applied with patient being awake until impedance increases i.e., when the coagulum is formed. The duration would usually be less than 1 minute. Sometimes, patient could even hear the crackling sound when the coagulum is made. In an in vitro study by Staudt MD, *et al.* in Operative Neurosurgery found that smaller power, longer duration, closer distance, bipolar thermocoagulation form a larger lesion [20].

### 3.2 Outcomes

In the systematic review of Pierre B, *et al.* in Epilepsia in 2018, six retrospective studies and 296 patients were included. Permanent neurological deficit was charted in 2.5% patients. Seizure-free outcome was achieved in average 23% while seizure response rate was up to 58% [21]. Greatest efficacy was observed in periventricular nodular heterotopia while lowest in non-lesional cases. Studies showed high heterogeneity concerning case selection and, therefore factors for good outcome are still unknown.

In the cohort study done by Alexis Moles, *et al.* in 2018, patients with temporal epilepsy with SEEG done was selected to the group of anterior temporal lobectomy and RFA as what procedure the patient had undergone. Three-quarters of patients in lobectomy group achieve seizure freedom in contrast to 0% in the RFA group [22]. Yet around half of the patients in the RFA were responder with no memory impairment recorded. In the cohort, SEEG-RFA is the first choice of treatment after SEEG implantation in the patients who were enrolled later after this treatment policy is employed. They would perform anterior temporal lobectomy if there is failure of the RFA and this would regard as treatment failure. So, the difference in the treatment outcome is not due to the different characteristics, but the treatment per se. Therefore, SEEG-RFA for temporal epilepsy could never achieve the same outcome as the well-established anterior temporal lobectomy and amygdalohippocampectomy but could offer some improvement in seizure control in the patients where lobectomy is contraindicated e.g., temporal lobe epilepsy in dominant hemisphere, apart from directly subjecting patients to neuromodulation. The target of this treatment is the ictal onset zone identified in the SEEG recordings instead of dealing with the entire EZ.

## 4. Brain-computer interface

Brain-computer interface (BCI) is a rapidly developing field in neuroscience. One area would the neuroprosthesis which receives electrical signals from the brain and perform tasks that patients with neurological deficits are not able do e.g., speech and movement. The hardware to receive the electrical signals include scalp EEG, ECoG and, of course, SEEG. Motor imagery, P300 and steady-state visual evoked potential (SSVEP) are some of the types of BCI [23]. Motor neuroprosthesis is the one that is better developed but recently the study by Moses DA, *et al.* showed the possibility of decoding the brain speech areas and produce speech for patient who was anarthric for a long time [24].

Currently scalp EEG and ECoG are the mainstay. However, like presurgical workup in epilepsy, SEEG provides a network analysis not only including the superficial structures but also the deep structures. It also provides a spatial and temporal appreciation of the electrical signals. Most importantly, it has a lower hemorrhagic or infective complication rates as compared with craniotomy. It probably leads to fewer gliosis as compared with subdural grid and provides better longevity. When the technology improves, the diameter of the electrodes as well as the intervals between electrodes become smaller [25]. The in vivo implantation could likely be successful as what functional neurosurgeons had been doing in deep brain stimulation.

## Author details

See Ka Wing Michael
Department of Neurosurgery, Queen Elizabeth Hospital, Hong Kong

*Address all correspondence to: drmichaelsee@gmail.com

## References

[1] Mullin JP, Smithason S, Gonzalez-Martinez J. Stereo-electro-encephalography (SEEG) with robotic assistance in the presurgical evaluation of medical refractory epilepsy: A technical note. Journal of Visualized Experiments. 2016;**112**:53206. DOI: 10.3791/53206

[2] Bancaud J, Talairach J, Bresson M, et al. Epileptic attacks induced by stimulation of the amygdaloid nucleus and horn of Ammon (value of stimulation in the determination of temporal epilepsy in humans). Revue Neurologique (Paris). 1968;**118**(6):527-532

[3] Khoo HM, Hall JA, Dubeau F, Tani N, Oshino S, Fujita Y, et al. Technical aspects of SEEG and its interpretation in the delineation of the epileptogenic zone. Neurologia Medico-Chirurgica (Tokyo). 2020;**60**(12):565-580. DOI: 10.2176/nmc.st.2020-0176

[4] Catenoix H, Bourdillon P, Guénot M, Isnard J. The combination of stereo-EEG and radiofrequency ablation. Epilepsy Research. 2018 May;**142**:117-120. DOI: 10.1016/j.eplepsyres.2018.01.012

[5] Kwan P, Arzimanoglou A, Berg AT, Brodie MJ, Allen Hauser W, Mathern G, et al. Definition of drug resistant epilepsy: Consensus proposal by the ad hoc Task Force of the ILAE Commission on therapeutic strategies. Epilepsia. 2010;**51**:1069-1077. DOI: 10.1111/j.1528-1167.2009.02397.x

[6] Obeid M, Wyllie E, Rahi AC, Mikati MA. Approach to pediatric epilepsy surgery: State of the art, Part I: General principles and presurgical workup. European Journal of Paediatric Neurology. 2009;**13**(2):102-114. ISSN 1090-3798. DOI: 10.1016/j.ejpn.2008.05.007

[7] Téllez-Zenteno JF, Hernández Ronquillo L, Moien-Afshari F, Wiebe S. Surgical outcomes in lesional and non-lesional epilepsy: A systematic review and meta-analysis. Epilepsy Research. 2010;**89**(2-3):310-318. DOI: 10.1016/j.eplepsyres.2010.02.007. Epub 2010 Mar 15

[8] Phal PM, Usmanov A, Nesbit GM, Anderson JC, Spencer D, Wang P, et al. Qualitative comparison of 3-T and 1.5-T MRI in the evaluation of epilepsy. American Journal of Roentgenology. 2008;**191**(3):890-895

[9] Poon TL. Presurgical evaluation of epilepsy surgery. In: Epilepsy - Update on Classification, Etiologies, Instrumental Diagnosis and Treatment. London: IntechOpen; 2020. DOI: 10.5772/intechopen.93602

[10] Catapano JS, Whiting AC, Wang DJ, Hlubek RJ, Labib MA, Morgan CD, et al. Selective posterior cerebral artery amobarbital test: A predictor of memory following subtemporal selective amygdalohippocampectomy. Journal of Neurointerventional Surgery. 2020;**12**(2):165-169. DOI: 10.1136/neurintsurg-2019-014984. Epub 2019 Jul 18

[11] Minotti L, Montavont A, Scholly J, Tyvaert L, Taussig D. Indications and limits of stereoelectroencephalography (SEEG). Neurophysiologie Clinique. 2018;**48**(1):15-24. ISSN 0987-7053. DOI: 10.1016/j.neucli.2017.11.006

[12] McGonigal A, Bartolomei F, Régis J, Guye M, Gavaret M, Trébuchon-Da Fonseca A, et al. Stereoelectroencephalography in presurgical assessment of MRI-negative epilepsy. Brain. 2007;**130**(Pt 12):3169-3183. DOI: 10.1093/brain/awm218. Epub 2007 Sep 12

[13] Mullin JP, Shriver M, Alomar S, Najm I, Bulacio J, Chauvel P, et al. Is SEEG safe? A systematic review and meta-analysis of stereo-electroencephalography-related complications. Epilepsia. 2016;**57**(3): 386-401. DOI: 10.1111/epi.13298. Epub 2016 Feb 21

[14] Arya R, Mangano FT, Horn PS, Holland KD, Rose DF, Glauser TA. Adverse events related to extraoperative invasive EEG monitoring with subdural grid electrodes: A systematic review and meta-analysis. Epilepsia. 2013;**54**:828-839. DOI: 10.1111/epi.12073

[15] Isnard J, Taussig D, Bartolomei F, Bourdillon P, Catenoix H, Chassoux F, et al. French guidelines on stereo-electroencephalography (SEEG). Neurophysiologie Clinique. 2018;**48**(1): 5-13. DOI: 10.1016/j.neucli.2017.11.005. Epub 2017 Dec 23

[16] Katz JS, Abel TJ. Stereoelectroencephalography versus subdural electrodes for localization of the epileptogenic zone: What is the evidence? Neurotherapeutics. 2019;**16**(1):59-66. DOI: 10.1007/s13311-018-00703-2

[17] Vakharia VN, Sparks R, O'Keeffe AG, Rodionov R, Miserocchi A, McEvoy A, et al. Accuracy of intracranial electrode placement for stereoencephalography: A systematic review and meta-analysis. Epilepsia. 2017;**58**(6):921-932. DOI: 10.1111/epi.13713. Epub 2017 Mar 6

[18] George DD, Ojemann SG, Drees C, Thompson JA. Stimulation mapping using stereoelectroencephalography: Current and future directions. Frontiers in Neurology. 2020;**11**:320. DOI: 10.3389/fneur.2020.00320

[19] Poon TL, Lui CHT, Chan I, Siu DYW. Updated review: Drug-resistant epilepsy and presurgical evaluation of epilepsy surgery. Hong Kong Medical Journal. 2018;**24**(6):610-616. Epub 27 Nov 2018. DOI: 10.12809/hkmj187285

[20] Staudt MD, Maturu S, Miller JP. Radiofrequency energy and electrode proximity influences stereoelectroencephalography-guided radiofrequency thermocoagulation lesion size: An in vitro study with clinical correlation. Operative Neurosurgery (Hagerstown, Md.). 2018;**15**(4):461-469. DOI: 10.1093/ons/opx291

[21] Bourdillon P, Cucherat M, Isnard J, Ostrowsky-Coste K, Catenoix H, Guénot M, et al. Stereo-electroencephalography-guided radiofrequency thermocoagulation in patients with focal epilepsy: A systematic review and meta-analysis. Epilepsia. 2018;**59**(12):2296-2304. DOI: 10.1111/epi.14584. Epub 2018 Oct 21

[22] Moles A, Guénot M, Rheims S, Berthiller J, Catenoix H, Montavont A, et al. SEEG-guided radiofrequency coagulation (SEEG-guided RF-TC) versus anterior temporal lobectomy (ATL) in temporal lobe epilepsy. Journal of Neurology. 2018;**265**(9):1998-2004. DOI: 10.1007/s00415-018-8958-9. Epub 2018 Jun 26

[23] Amiri S, Rabbi A, Azinfar L, Fazel-Rezai R. A review of P300, SSVEP, and hybrid P300/SSVEP brain-computer interface systems. In: Brain-Computer Interface Systems - Recent Progress and Future Prospects. London: IntechOpen; 2013. DOI: 10.5772/56135

[24] Moses DA, Metzger SL, Liu JR, Anumanchipalli GK, Makin JG, Sun PF, et al. Neuroprosthesis for decoding speech in a paralyzed person with Anarthria. The New England Journal of Medicine. 2021;**385**(3):217-227. DOI: 10.1056/NEJMoa2027540

[25] Herff C, Krusienski DJ, Kubben P. The potential of stereotactic-EEG for brain-computer interfaces: Current progress and future directions. Frontiers in Neuroscience. 2020;**14**:123. DOI: 10.3389/fnins.2020.00123

Chapter 5

# Recent Advances in Epilepsy Surgery

*Ahmad Tamimi, Malik Juweid and Iskandar Tamimi*

## Abstract

The modern practice of epilepsy surgery requires multiple modalities of presurgical investigations such as video-EEG, intracranial EEG, high-resolution imaging, advanced functional imaging, and clinical analysis. A multidisciplinary approach is essential, including close collaboration between neurosurgeons, neurologists, neurophysiologists, neuropsychologists, neuropsychiatrists, and neuroradiologists. Candidates for epilepsy surgery require a history of seizures that are refractory to appropriate medical therapy. A meticulous selection of candidates will lead to a better chance of freedom from seizure. Epilepsy surgery includes a variety of surgical procedures including resective surgery for focal refractory seizure, which offers a significant chance of seizure freedom in temporal and extratemporal lobe epilepsy. Palliative treatment for patients who are not candidates for resective surgery, such as vagal nerve stimulation, deep stimulation, and callosotomy, offers further options. We reviewed and analyzed the recent scientific literature and forthcoming advances that will impact on the future of epilepsy surgery. This chapter on recent advances in epilepsy surgery emphasizes improved methods of assessment, a better understanding of seizures, the development of new surgical techniques, and the outcome of epilepsy surgery.

**Keywords:** epilepsy, refractory seizure, surgery, temporal lobe epilepsy, vagus nerve stimulation, callostomy, recent advances

## 1. Introduction

Epilepsy is a brain disorder characterized by brief disturbances in the normal electrical function of the brain resulting in seizures; 35% of adults with active epilepsy have seizures that are not seen by a neurologist or an epilepsy specialist [1].

Epilepsy is one of the most common chronic neurologic disorders with a worldwide prevalence of approximately 1.2% [2]. Epilepsy contributes to up to 25% of the global burden of neurological disease, and many neurological diseases are associated with seizures and epilepsy [3].

Recent data indicate that epilepsy mortality rates are rising significantly [4]. These data have generated significant concern from stakeholders and advocacy groups that the increase in epilepsy mortality may represent a failure to effectively treat epilepsy and prevent premature death [5].

Only 64% of patients with new-onset seizures are seizure-free by their third anti-epileptic drugs (AED) [6]. Thus, more than 35% of patients continue to have seizures and become recognized as refractory seizure patients.

The pre-surgical evaluation should result in a clear understanding of whether surgery can be undertaken and its potential benefit [7].

Neuroimaging developments with the introduction of magnetic resonance imaging (MRI), functional (fMRI), fluourodeoxyglucose F18 positron emission tomography (PET), single-photon emission computed tomography (SPECT), and magnetoencephalography (MEG) have facilitated the selection of patients for surgery, also reducing the number and severity of complications [8, 9]. Neurophysiological tests include invasive and noninvasive procedures and define the epileptogenic zone in a specialized center. Epilepsy surgery should be recommended through a multidisciplinary team [5].

In pharmacoresistant (PR) patients, epilepsy surgery must take into consideration the chance of seizure freedom and the adverse long-term effects of uncontrolled seizures [10]. Epilepsy surgery is underutilized even in developed countries because many physicians do not recognize that a treatable syndrome exists and in developing countries because of lack of resources or because many physicians do not recognize that a treatable syndrome exists [5].

Developments made in surgical techniques have significantly increased the effectiveness and safety of these techniques as such techniques have been demonstrated to improve seizure control/freedom outcomes [11] and increase patients' life span [8] by reducing the number and severity of complications [8, 9].

## 2. Refractory seizure

One percent of the world's population has active epilepsy, 30–40% of people with epilepsy have a seizure that is uncontrolled by medication [1], which accounts for 80% of the cost of epilepsy in the United States [12].

PR epilepsy is, therefore, a major health concern for patients, their families, and for the society. Treatment aim for epilepsy is seizure freedom with no side effects, as soon as possible. Full-service epilepsy centers are staffed by a multidisciplinary team consisting of neurologists, epileptologist, neurosurgeons, neuroradiologists, clinical neurophysiologists, neuropsychologists, psychiatrists, social workers, and nurses skilled in the management of epileptic seizures and their consequences [13]. These approaches permit recognition of true epileptic seizures and their causes, diagnosis of specific seizure types and epilepsy syndromes, and determination of which patients are truly FRs and might be candidates for surgical therapy.

Apparent pharmacotherapy failure does not necessarily mean that standard AEDs will not work. Alternative causes are seizures that are not epileptic, misdiagnosis of the seizure type or epilepsy syndrome, inappropriate use of AED such as inadequate doses or drug interactions and lifestyle issues, such as drug abuse, alcohol binging, stress, and sleep deprivation. Epilepsy centers have the ability to utilize specialized pharmacologic approaches, including enrollment in clinical trials of experimental anti-seizure drugs, to provide alternative treatments other than surgery,

The term "PR epilepsy" can no longer be taken literally, as there are now so many anti-seizure drugs that it would take a lifetime to try all of them alone and in combination in any given patient.

There are several reasons for PR, and research to clarify underlying mechanisms is important for the future development for more effective treatments [14].

Concerning the diagnosis of PR patients, the International League Against Epilepsy (ILAE) has proposed, as a verifiable hypothesis: "That PR is defined as failure of adequate trials of two tolerated, appropriately selected, and used antiepileptic drug schedules (monotherapies or in combination) to achieve sustained seizure freedom, which is defined as sustaining seizure freedom for a period 3 times the longest inter-seizure interval or 1 year whichever is longer" [15].

## 3. Epileptogenic zone

The epileptogenic zone is defined as the area of the cortex that is necessary and sufficient for initiating seizures and whose removal 0r disconnection is necessary for the complete abolition of seizures [16].

The pre-surgical evaluation to define the epileptogenic zone and its relationship with the eloquent area is essential for the ideal resection for a patient with drug-resistant focal epilepsy (**Figure 1**) [8].

Jehi [17] defined five cortical zones in the pre-surgical evaluation process, which include: the irrigative zone (IZ), which is the area of the cortex that generates electric spikes, with the best test to define that through EEG, MEG and EEG-fMRI; seizure onset zone (SOZ), which is that area of the cortex responsible of the clinical seizure tested by EEG, ictal SPECT, fMRI, and MEG; symptomatic zone (SZ), defined as the area of the cortex that, when activated produces initial ictal symptoms signs, observed by initial seizure symptomology; epileptogenic lesion (EL) includes macroscopic lesion that is causative of the epileptic seizure because the lesion itself is epileptogenic (cortical dysplasia) by secondary hyperexcitability of the adjacent cortex, tested by MRI; functional deficit zone (FDZ) defined as the area of the cortex that is not functioning normally in the inter-ictal period tested by neurological and psychological exams and by functional images (interictal SPECT and PET) (**Table 1**).

It is helpful in the study of epileptogenic zone to use intracranial EEG (subdural electrode or SDE implantation via craniotomy) as a principal approach for intracranial EEG monitoring [18]. Nevertheless, there is no high-quality evidence indicating superiority of any one technique over the other intracranial EEG monitoring [19],

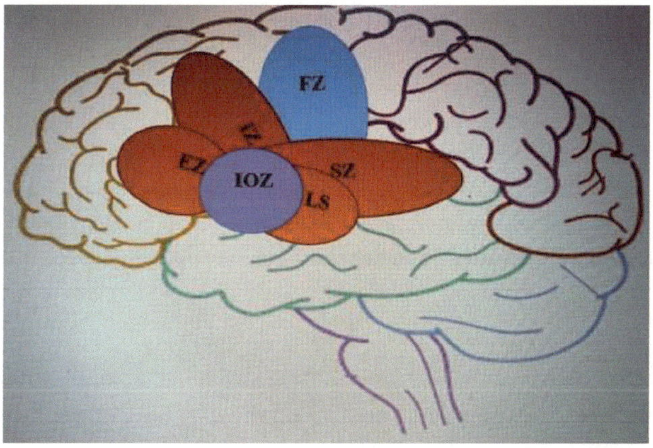


**Figure 1.**
*Epileptogenic complex cortical area. IOZ; ictal onset zone, IZ; Irritative zone, FZ; functional zone, SZ; symptomatogenic zone, EZ; epileptogenic zone, LS; lesion area.*

| Critical zone | Diagnostic procedures |
|---|---|
| Functional deficit zone; area of the cortex with abnormal function in the intricately period | Clinical neurological and neuropsychological examination. PET and Inter ictal SPECT |
| Epileptogenic lesion area; were the lesion is responsible of the seizure, such as migratory disorders. | Brain MRI |
| Symptomatic zone; are of the cortex that that during seizure activation produce symptoms or signs. | Clinical initial seizure and Video EEG |
| Seizure onset zone; area of the cortex the initiate the clinical seizures | Video EEG, Ictal SPECT |
| Irritative zone: area of the cortex that generate inter ictal spikes | EEG, MEG, EEG-fMRI |
| Epileptogenic network | Micro dialysis; (Glutamate level at onset of seizure and in epileptogenic region) |
| | 7TMR spectroscopy image(spectrometer); mainly in medical temporal lobe epilepsy) MTLE and MTS. |
| | Neurotransmitters; Central benzodiazepine receptors acts on ionotropic $GABA_A$–regulation in seizure complex, which is reduced in epileptogenic foci and seizure onset. |
| | Dopamine receptor; Dopamine receptor D2/D3 decrease in epileptogenic area(PET) Opioid receptors, trough PET radiotracers, no changes in temporal lobe epilepsy. |
| Tractography | Difussion tensor imaging(DTI), can visualizeze Meyer Loop preoperativly. |

**Table 1.**
*Preoperative evaluation modalities for delimitation of epilepsy zone in refractory seizure patients.*

specific brain MRI with sequence and voxel-based morphometric analysis, and the EEG-fMRI [20]. 3D multimodality images are a simultaneous display of different structural and functional data in each patient [17–19].

Unidentified epileptogenic source occurs in approximately 50% of patients coming to surgery [21]. According to advanced knowledge in EZ, defining the area of neuro-connectivity through the epileptogenic network is very important. This is achieved by using new tests for epileptogenic network detection: a) microanalysis; by detecting the extracellular glutamate level, through microanalysis device insertion; glutamate level is increased in the epileptogenic region and high at onset of seizure [22]. b) 7 T-MR spectroscopy, in the study of mesiotemporal lobe sclerosis (MTLS), the epileptogenic in the hippocampus is energetically developed, anterior more than posterior; a similar energetic loss is seen in the ipsilateral anterior thalamus and less significantly in the contralateral thalamus and hippocampus [23]. According to this, optogenetic stimulation of thalamic circuit can inhibit the parietal epileptogenic cortex.

## 4. Presurgical evaluation

The pre-surgical evaluation is the most crucial aspect for epilepsy surgery; all patients diagnosed with PR should be referred to an epilepsy center for pre-surgical evaluation to confirm the diagnosis of true epilepsy and type of seizure. At this stage of evaluation, around 50% of patients usually have idiopathic generalized seizure, which cannot be treated with resective epilepsy surgery; only patients with focal-onset seizure with loss of awareness (partial complex seizure) with or without secondary generalized seizure are surgical candidates and can complete the pre-surgical process for investigation. Therefore, the initial evaluation should include proper history, seizure semiology, and EEG. The final goal of pre-surgical evaluation is to define the EZ (region) defining the lateralization and localization of EZ (**Table 2**) [24].

The American Epilepsy Society conference had a consensus about the evaluation protocol through a multidisciplinary methodological approach involving physical exam, scalp video-EEG, telemetry, structural MRI (MRI epilepsy protocol), neuropsychological assessment, neuropsychiatric assessment, social worker, and nursing for patient support network, with realistic expectation of outcome [25]. Additionally parameters include fMRI, Wada test, PET, ictal SPECT, MEG, and intracranial EEG electrodes (**Table 1**) [25, 26].

### 4.1 Neurological and neuropsychological studies

Neurological and neuropsychological assessment is part of the preoperative evaluation of refractory seizure patients. The assessment should comprise baseline standardized measures of cognitive function in addition to wider measures of behavioral

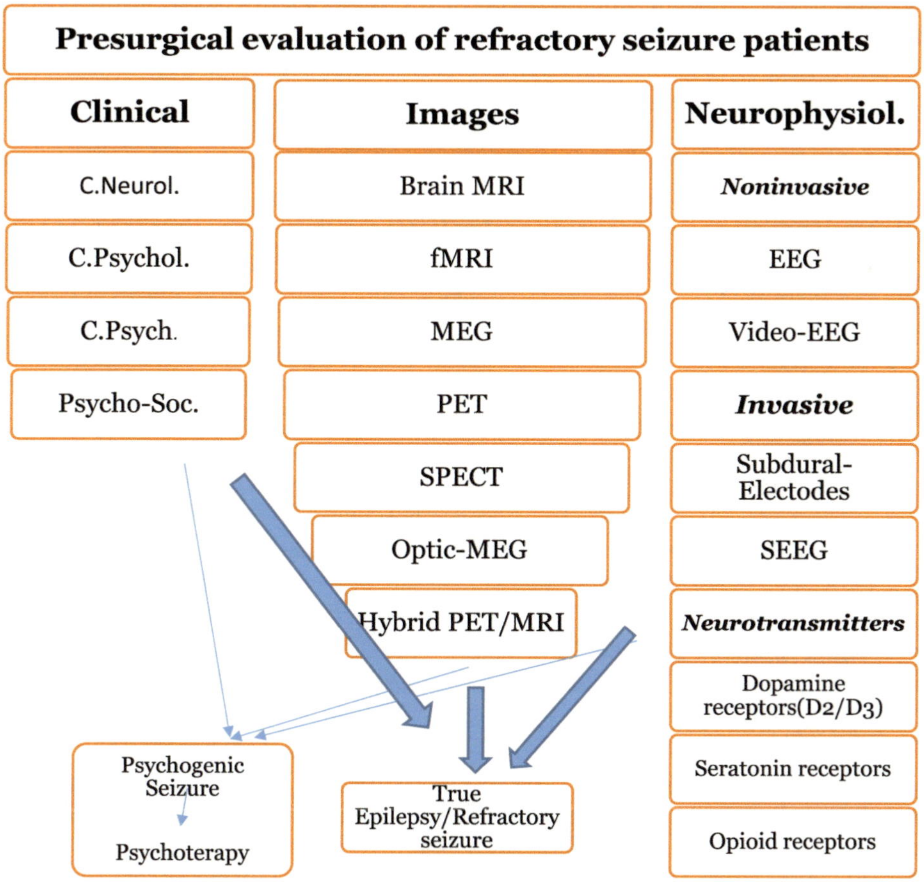


**Table 2.**
*Pre-surgical evaluation parameters of patients with refractory seizure.*

and psychosocial function [27]. The preoperative neuropsychological assessment contributes to seizure lateralization, localization, characterization, and provides predictions of cognitive risk associated with surgery [27].

For future outcome, it is important to include exploration of patient and family expectations from surgical treatment. Neuropsychological changes following surgery are a dynamic process, and it should be an integral part of the postoperative follow-up. The neuropsychologist plays an important role with postoperative rehabilitation and support of the patient and family members as a part of the multidisciplinary team of epilepsy surgery [28].

## 4.2 Electrophysiological studies

### *4.2.1 Noninvasive EEG monitoring*

The standard procedure after confirming PR patient usually is initiated with video EEG-monitoring for detection of lateralization and localization of seizure focus. Patients are often admitted for several days, depending on their seizure frequency. Most often their AEDs are tapered off in order to capture about 3–5 typical and consistent seizures. There is no consensus on the tapering process, but in general very rapid tapering is avoided to minimize risk of status epilepticus or triggering aberrant seizure onset zones [24, 29].

Scalp-recorded EEG is usually performed for inter-ictal and ictal epileptiform patterns [29]. In the video-EEG monitoring, seizure semiology is recorded, which is important for surgical decision-making [29]. Occasionally when ictal/inter-ictal EEG epileptiform activity discharges are concordant with structural neuroimaging abnormalities, it could be sufficient for surgical localization and treatment [26]. High-density array of EEG electrodes (10–10 electrode placement) may be useful in patient with extra-temporal lobe focal seizure. Deeper seizure foci may not be detected via (scalp) electrodes. Further, scalp EEG recording is usually insufficient in extra-temporal epilepsy or even in non-lesional (normal MRI) temporal lobe epilepsy (TLE). Using extra electrodes placed based on the 10–10 international electrode system may add significant accuracy to scalp recording and in some cases avoid intracranial recording [24].

When seizure onset zone is poorly lateralized due to alternating seizure onset lateralization in bi-temporal asynchrony or frequent bilateral epileptiform discharges, it indicates a less favorable postsurgical seizure outcome [30]. Unilateral hippocampal atrophy on MRI and concordant unilateral interictal spikes are highly predictive of concordant ictal localization [31].

### *4.2.2 Invasive intracranial EEG*

ECoG, implantation of SDE, is very helpful in detecting, seizure lateralization and localization. The duration of intra cranial-EEG monitoring is determined by seizure frequency, number of seizures needed to make a decision, and the time needed to perform mapping of the eloquent cortex. Interpretation of the data is based on EEG pattern recognition as well as clinical semiology.

It is essential to insert the intracranial EEG electrodes in proper locations at or in close vicinity to the epileptogenic zone although interpretation may be difficult in some cases since that frequency range may differ from one cerebral area to another due to neurophysiological properties of the anatomical structure and from one etiology to another [24, 32].

*4.2.3 Stereoelectroencephalography (SEEG)*

Recording EEG signals through surgically implanted depth electrodes provides the best coverage for deeper structures (such as hippocampus, amygdala, and insula) and deep sulci. Depth electrodes in various lengths and number of contacts are implanted using conventional stereotactic technique or by the assistance of stereotactic robotic devices through 2.5 mm diameter drill holes. Risk of infection and intracranial hemorrhage have been reported in 1% of patients. In other series small hemorrhages have been reported in 5.5%, of whom only 0.9% required surgery, and no mortality was reported [33, 34]. The planning of SEEG implantation requires formulating precise hypotheses about the possible epileptogenic zone, seizure onset, and propagation zones to be tested.

### 4.3 Neuroimaging studies

Advances in brain imaging technology have substantially improved seizure localization and surgical outcome [30]. All patients with clinical and evidence of focal-onset seizure should have brain imaging, including brain MRI [24].

*4.3.1 Brain MRI*

MRI is an important noninvasive tool for evaluation of patient with epilepsy that provides two critical data, a potential epileptogenic brain abnormality, and its surrounded anatomy. Whole brain coverage allows for the examination of the lesion location and its relationship to cortical eloquent areas [35]. The main role of brain MRI is to define structural abnormalities that may cause seizure. A high-resolution brain MRI, with epilepsy protocol, is recommended. Epileptogenic lesions in almost one half of those presenting with new-onset seizure are detected. Sensitivity of brain MRI is increased by using epilepsy protocol [36]. The common sequences used by most epilepsy centers include thin section of 1 mm coronal oblique T1 gradient echo, coronal oblique T2 series, high-resolution 3D sequences (sensitive to subtle cortical dysplasia or small tumors), and T2 flair (fluid attenuated inversion recovery) images performed on 3 Tesla or higher MRI systems [24].

*4.3.2 Functional brain MRI (fMRI)*

The functional MRI acquisitions are based on the blood oxygen level dependent (BOLD), the main target is to confirm language hemisphere dominance in patients that are candidates for possible temporal lobe resection. It has been widely used in the context of pre-surgical evaluation in refractory seizure, is a noninvasive procedure, and is able to provide more precise localization and more cost-effective than the invasive Wada Test (with intracarotid amobarbital injection [25]. According to the American Academy of Neurology, fMRI, it is part of the guideline for language and memory function and should be predicting postoperative verbal memory outcome [37]. It can be also used in mapping of primary motor, somatosensory cortex, or visual cortex, which is useful for certain tumors, gliosis, or focal cortical dysplasia, with close relationship to eloquent area [31]. EEG-fMRI may yield complementary information within the pre-surgical evaluation for patients with possible surgical treatment [36].

#### *4.3.3 Magnetoencephalography (MEG)*

MEG is a noninvasive functional neuroimaging method for investigating electrical neuronal activity of the living human brain by using sensors positioned around the head [38] that measure fluxes in the magnetic field caused by the same brain electrical activity, which is excellent for spatial and temporal resolution and is complementary to scalp EEG [38]. However, certain limitation for the wide use of MEG is due to signal disturbance caused by subject motion and the high maintenance cost [38].

#### *4.3.4 Optic-magnetoencephalography (OP-MEG)*

This method functions through optic-pumped magnetometers and high Tc SQUIDs and does not require a thermal isolation [39]. It allows to move the subject naturally while recording long-term OP-MEG recording akin to EEG telemetry, which is especially useful in pediatric epilepsy [39].

#### *4.3.5 Single photon emission computerized tomography (SPECT)*

This functional neuroimaging modality is based on a radioactive tracer, imaging hardware, and data analysis software. $^{99m}$Tc-ethyl cysteinate dimmer [ECD or Neurolyte$^{R}$] or $^{99m}$Tc-99 m HMPAO SPECT is used for measurement of regional cerebral blood flow in vivo [40]. Compared with $^{18}$F-FDG PET, brain SPECT has inferior spatial but superior temporal resolution, allowing identification of onset-zone and increased neuronal activity during the ictal phase, which is associated with increased metabolism and regional cerebral blood flow (RCBF) [40]. SPECT can also detect additional abnormalities in regions without structural abnormalities.

#### *4.3.6 Fluorodeoxyglucose positron emission tomography (FDG-PET)*

FDG-PET is an indirect marker of neuronal energy metabolism by measurement of glucose consumption. PET is obtained during the inter-ictal phase because cerebral uptake of FDG occurs over 30–40 minutes after injection and represents the imaging consumption of cellular metabolic process during the uptake period. The prolonged cerebral metabolic uptake makes FDG inappropriate for measuring rapid neural events considering the average seizure duration of 1–2 minutes; thus, ictal FDG PET is not usually feasible [40, 41]. Epileptogenic foci of inter-ictal TLE and extra TLE are associated with the area of reduced glucose metabolism that usually extends beyond the seizure-onset zone [30].

#### *4.3.7 Hybrid PET/MRI*

PET/MRI has shown improved diagnostic yields in detecting potential epileptogenic lesions in patients with refractory seizures presenting for possible epilepsy surgery [42]. The choice of tracer depends on the physiological process of interest such as oxygen consumption, glucose metabolism, or cerebral blood flow. The sensitivity of detecting unilateral temporal lobe hypometabolism by inter-ictal FDG-PET/MRI is 70–80% [42].

*4.3.8 Non-FDG PET procedures (neurotransmitters)*

*4.3.8.1 Central benzodiazepine receptors*

Carbon-11-labeled Flumazenil (FMZ) is a specific reversible bound antagonist to the central benzodiazepine site on the $GABA_A$ receptor complex. GABA receptor binding and FMZ uptake are reduced in the epileptogenic foci, and the seizure onset zone has narrower distribution than the corresponding area of FDG hypometabolism. However, an area of focal decrease of FMZ uptake in the cortical regions remote from the primary focus may occur complicating localization of epileptogenic focus [43].

*4.3.8.2 Dopamine receptors*

Awareness of dopamine role in the pathophysiology of focal epilepsy is growing after the discovery of dopamine receptors (D1, D2, D3); D1 more pro-convulsant, and D2s have anticonvulsant effect [4, 44]. PET studies with the high affinity of D2/D3 receptors radioligand $^{18}$F-fallypride have shown that D2/D3 receptor levels are significantly decreased in the epileptogenic temporal lobe in all patients, including the temporal pole and lateral temporal region in patients with TLE and hippocampal sclerosis, which inhibit decreased FDG uptake. These findings suggest that dopaminergic system is part of the endogenous anticonvulsant mechanism that prevents generalization of the seizure [44].

*4.3.8.3 Serotonin receptors*

PET radio-tracer $^{11}$C-α- methyl- tryptophan (AMT) is used for quantification of serotonin synthesis in the brain, which is increased in cortex epileptic area and reveals the epileptogenic focus in the inter-ictal state [44].

*4.3.8.4 Opioid receptors*

Functional imaging with PET radiotracers yields quantitative measurement of opioid binding mediated by μ, γ κ, opioid receptors. This has not demonstrated specific changes in TLE idiopathic epilepsy [4].

## 5. Surgical approaches and techniques

Surgery is an effective procedure for many patients with drug-resistant epilepsy (DRE). Unfortunately, surgery is underutilized; in the USA, <1% of patients with DRE are referred to epilepsy centers [45]. The common reasons for rejections include fear of complications, expenses, reservation about benefits, and misconceptions held by non-specialist physicians [6, 45]. The delay from onset of epilepsy to surgery averages >20 years resulting in impaired social and educational development [8]. Early surgery provides the best opportunity for seizure remission minimizing adverse social and psychological consequences and premature death [6].

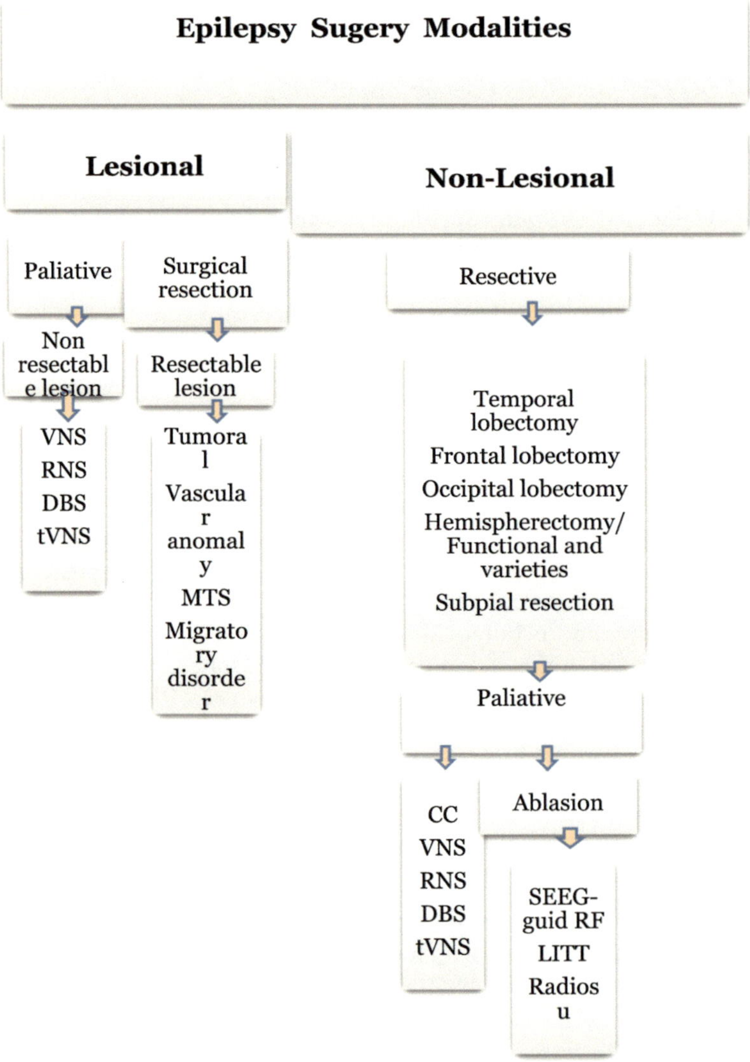


**Table 3.**
*Epilepsy surgery, modalities according to the preoperative evaluation.*

Surgical therapy can eliminate disabling seizures completely in appropriately selected patients [46]. Multiple surgical procedures, including recent minimally invasive procedures, are now offered depending on the type of epileptic seizures and their presumed underling pathology (**Table 3**).

### 5.1 General anesthetic consideration

Perioperative anxiety should be managed with premedication in the preoperative area. Midazolam has been demonstrated to be effective in relieving anxiety. If intra-operative ECoG is planed the dosage of Midazolam and Benzodiazepines should be reduced to minimize their depression effect on ECoG intraoperatively [47].

Anesthesia can be induced with thiopental or Propofol; these drugs rapidly induce the unconsciousness nondepolarizing muscle relaxant in the administration after induction of general anesthesia [47].

### 5.2 Awake anesthesia in epilepsy surgery

The golden rule in epilepsy surgery is to resect the epileptogenic zone, with preservation of the neurological function [48]. The epileptogenic zone often shows no image abnormalities (FCD type I) in foci often located in functional areas, such as language or somatosensory areas. In such situations, awake surgery may be effective [48]. The main advantage of awake anesthesia is the clinical functional mapping intraoperatively under awake condition allowing the identification of eloquent area with close monitoring during resection. Positioning the patient is critical for the success of the technique "Asleep-awake-asleep." Propofol does not interfere with ECoG monitoring when disconnected 20 minutes before [24]. Certain disadvantages have been reported, such as spatial limitation of craniotomy, limited intraoperative time, inability to have ictal recording, and limitation of the patient cooperation in young patients or patients with psychological or psychiatric disorders. However, in awake anesthesia, it is imperative to psychologically prepare the patient for the procedure. It has been reported that under awake anesthesia, patients with epileptogenic foci, close to functional area, may have improved seizure control and minimal neurological complications, through intraoperative mapping information and ECoG [48].

### 5.3 Implantation of strip, grid, and depth electrodes

Invasive monitoring tests are indicated in cases of nonconclusive noninvasive tests, with unclear lateralization or localization of the epileptogenic zone. Invasive monitoring is not an exploratory procedure, but it is a complementary test for lateralization and localization of the epileptogenic zone [49]. The most common electrodes are subdural strip and grids. Epidural electrodes are available but not widely used. The ideal electrode should be selected by epileptologist, epilepsy surgeon, and neurophysiologist together after review of the all patient data. Invasive electrodes are frequently placed bilaterally, if lateralization is unclear [50]. Strip and depth electrodes are useful for lateralization of seizure onset while grids are more helpful in localization.

Depth electrodes are more valuable for assessment of deep cortical structures, such as amygdala, hippocampus, insular, cingulum, and bifrontal cortex. They have multiple contact arrays, up to 12 nickel-chromium, or platinum contact and are commonly in use for bi-temporal mesial sclerosis, and it could be used in combination with subdural electrodes [51].

Subdural strip (**Figure 2a–c**) and grids (**Figure 2d**) are fine structures covered by silastic or Teflon sheets embedded in nickel-chromium or platinum. Each electrode is 2–4 mm contact in diameter with inter-electrode distance being generally 10 mm. Subdural grids are larger plates of rectangular arrays with several parallel rows up to 64 electrodes. It is an excellent choice for covering large cortical area to record inter ictal and ictal epileptogenic activity. Cortical stimulation and grid mapping are valuable to delineate the functional area and epileptogenic zone [52]. The most common complications are subdural hematoma, up to 16%, cerebral edema, (2–14%), CSF leakages (19–33%), brain edema, 2–14%, hemiparesis, 1.5% [52].

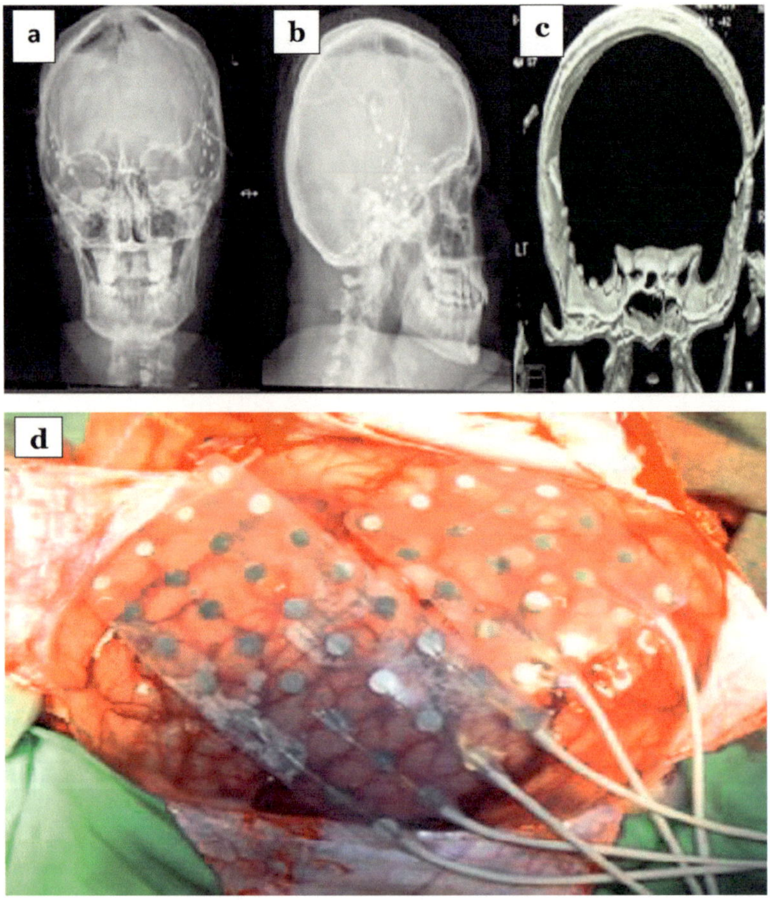


**Figure 2.**
*Intracranial monitoring; a & b; skull x-ray images, showing temporal bilateral intracranial strip electrodes, c; brain CT, axial cut, bone window technique, showing bilateral temporal intracranial electrodes. And d; intraoperative view showing over the brain cortex, 2 grids (4x8 &4x5 electrodes).*

## 5.4 Resective surgery for temporal lobe epilepsy

### *5.4.1 Temporal lobe epilepsy (TLE)*

TLE is the most common focal seizure disorder in adults with mesial temporal sclerosis being the most common pathological entity (10). Several varieties of techniques have been described, including tailored temporal lobectomy, anteromesial temporal lobectomy, trans-Sylvian amygdalohippocampectomy, and temporal lobe lesionectomy [53]. The overall seizure freedom following temporal lobectomy for epilepsy has been reported to be between 74 and 82%, with best outcome for temporal lobe neoplasm (88–92%), followed by patients with MTS (70%), and the poorest control for cortical dysplasia [54].

Resection of the anterior temporal lobe, the amygdala, and part of the hippocampus is the most commonly performed resective epilepsy surgery [55]. The posterior margin of resection is 4.0–4.5 cm in the dominant side, and 5.0–5.5 cm in the non-dominant hemisphere, in order to minimize the speech and visual deficits

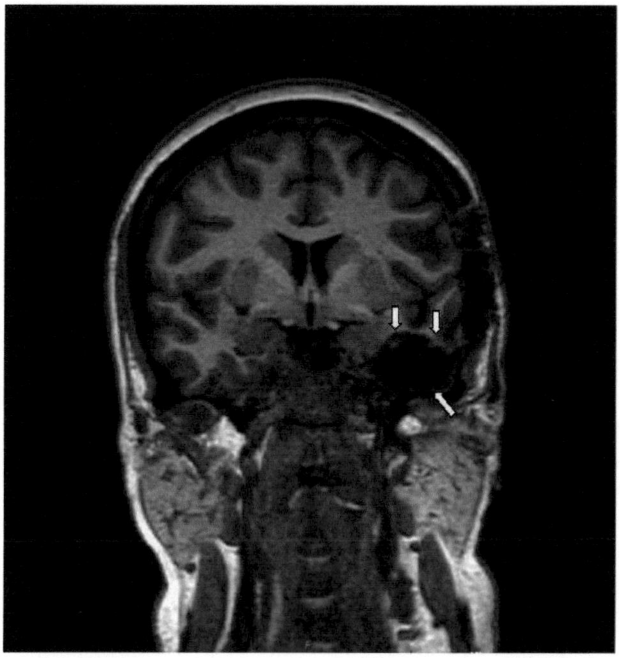

**Figure 3.**
*Brain MRI T1-weighted image, axial slide showing postsurgical temporal lobectomy and amygdalohypocampectomy.*

and an en bloc resection of the amygdala, hippocampus, uncus, and fusiform gyrus [56]. Schram et al. [57], in a review study of 53 scientific papers, showed no differences between temporal lobectomy and selective amygdala hippocampectomy. Nevertheless, neurophysiological outcome was significantly better in selective amygdalohippocampectomy [57]. Approximately 25% of patients will develop some degree of memory impairment after temporal lobe lobectomy (**Figure 3**) [55].

### *5.4.2 Resective surgery in extra-temporal lobe epilepsy*

Focal lesion, lobar or multilobar resections can be undertaken in the frontal, occipital, and parietal lobes with the expectation of curing or improving seizures. Lesions in eloquent areas of speech, language, and motor function may not be suitable for resection given the postoperative implications of this procedure. In areas adjacent to motor and somatosensory cortex, intraoperative neuro monitoring may be required. The outcomes of non-lesional or MRI-negative resections are less successful [55].

Most patients with extratemporal resections will have invasive electrode recordings because the epileptogenic zone is often not as well defined as in temporal-lobe epilepsy. The outcome for extra temporal-lobe resections is in the region of 60% [52]. Predictors of success include a greater extent of surgical resection, structural pathology on MRI, and concordant structural and electrophysiological imaging. For patients with cortical dysplasia, seizure freedom outcomes are reported to be in the region of 40–70% and are inversely related to the length of follow-up [58]. The best postoperative outcome is associated with type 2B focal cortical dysplasia [58].

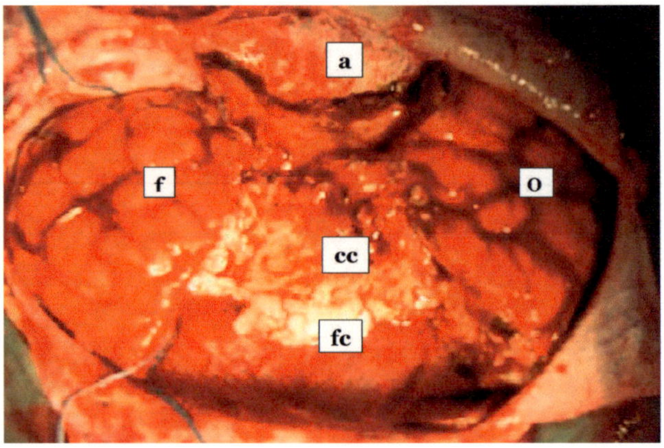


**Figure 4.**
*Intraoperative functional hemispherectomy view showing the middle cranial fossa after removal of the temporal lobe(a), falx cerebri (fc) and corpus callosum(cc) after removal of the parietal lobe, temporal lobectomy and disconnection of the frontal lobe(f), and occipital lobe(o).*

Frontal lobe resections account for up to 30% of cases and carry a 1-year seizure remission rate of approximately 45% (range 21–61%) and less durable long-term outcomes [59]. The EZ frequently extends beyond MRI-defined lesions, and the resection may need to be tailored according to invasive EEG findings [52]. The best postoperative outcome is associated with type 2B focal cortical dysplasia, a focal seizure onset, and total resection of the EZ.

In insular resection, seizure remission after resection of insular tumor is in the range of 74–84% [60], and insular resection with non-lesional requires a meticulous analysis of the risk–benefit ratio.

Usually parietal seizures are associated with lesional areas; seizure freedom ranges between 45 and 78%, with the best being associated with a focal MRI lesion [61]. Occipital lobe resection seizure freedom averages 65% (range between 52 and 100%) [61]. While occipital lobe epilepsy surgery carries significant risk of postoperative visual dysfunction, seizure freedom is less than that of frontal and parietal lobe.

### *5.4.3 Functional hemispherectomy*

When the EZ is extensive in one hemisphere, hemispherectomy, or functional hemispherectomy, may be considered. Generally, this is restricted to individuals who have a hemiparesis with loss of meaningful hand function [6]. Seizure freedom occurred in73% of patients. Most patients who are walking prior to surgery remain so afterward, whereas cognitive outcomes are usually stable, with language functions having developed in the contralateral hemisphere (**Figure 4**) [6].

## 6. Palliative treatment

### 6.1 Corpus callosotomy

This is a palliative interhemispheric surgical approach for PR patients, which consists of surgical disconnection of the corpus callosum to disrupt synchronization of epileptiform discharges between both brain hemispheres. It is indicated in multifocal ictal onset where seizures emanate from bilateral cortical foci at different frequency. Indication could also include failed or poor response with VNS implantation [62].

Concerning the outcome, several studies have suggested that complete corpus callosotomy is more effective, and its efficacy is sustainable with less relapse rates compared with anterior 2/3 corpus callosotomy (88% versus 58% in pediatric patients, [63]. Drop attacks improved from corpus callosotomy more than other generalized seizure types. Transient disconnection syndrome was significantly more likely in total corpus callosotomy than in anterior 2/3 corpus callosotomy [63, 64].

The decision whether to perform anterior 2/3 corpus callosotomy versus complete/ total corpus callosotomy is based on the degree of cognitive impairment and developmental delay and is also guided intraoperatively in some subjects by the presence of EEG activity desynchronization or transformation of generalized epileptiform

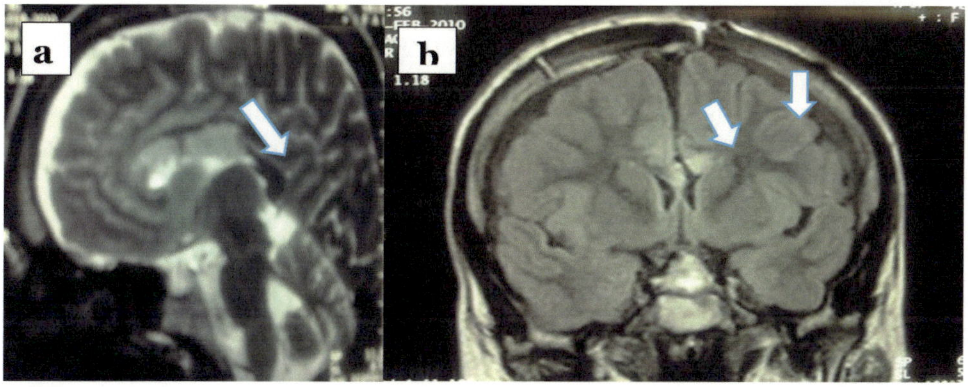


**Figure 5.**
*Corpus callosotomy; (a); brain MRI, coronal section T1 weighted, showing the disconnection of the corpus callosum (one row), (b); brain MRI sagittal section T2-weighted showing anterior 2/3 of the disconnection of the corpus callosum (2 rows).*

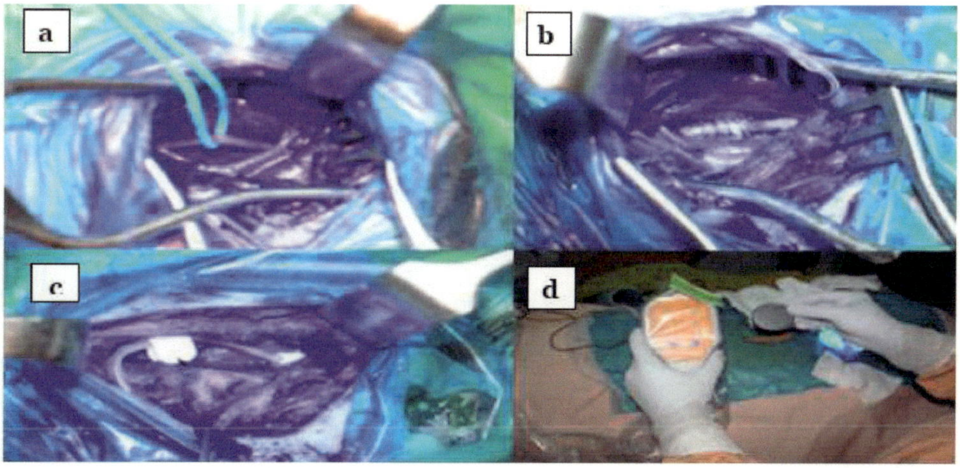


**Figure 6.**
*Vagus nerve insertion, a: Vagus nerve dissection, b: Electrode insertion, around the VNS, c: The lead of the device fixed to the muscle, and introduced subcutaneous to the infrascapular area, d: Intraoperative cheek of the stimulator, before subcutaneous insertion.*

discharges to asynchronized (lateralized) epileptiform discharges during the surgical course of the corpus callosotomy procedure (**Figure 5**) [64].

### 6.2 Vagus nerve stimulation

This is a type of stimulation of the vagus nerve on a set schedule. It is a well-established palliative treatment although it seems that VNS is unlikely to offer a substantial advance in epilepsy surgery. Current evidence points toward a deactivation of the nucleus of the solitary tract with widespread projections to the dorsal raphe nucleus, locus coerules, thalamus, hypothalamus, amygdala, and hippocampus [18]. A metanalysis has demonstrated a 44.1% decrease in seizure frequency with a follow-up of more than 3 years (**Figure 6**) [65].

### 6.3 Responsive neuro-stimulator (RNS)

RNS is a programmable neurostimulator, which is cranially implanted and connected to one or two depth and/or subdural cortical strip electrodes to detect the onset of seizure and stop it as it occurs. It is now gaining a major position in the USA as a new device with closed-loop system [66]. It is more effective in focal onset seizure, with 75% of seizure reduction [67].

### 6.4 Deep brain stimulation

This approach has attained approval as adjunctive therapy for refractory seizure in EU and USA [68]. Bilateral stimulation of the anterior nuclei of the thalamus (ANT) for epilepsy is indicated as an adjunctive therapy for reducing the frequency of seizure in adult patients with partial onset seizure with or without secondary generalized seizure [68]. The long-term data showed a median seizure reduction at 1 year of 41% increasing to 69% after 5 years [68]. The mechanism of action remains unknown. These modalities of adjunctive procedures are eventually available in most developed countries [69].

### 6.5 (t-VNS)

Transcutaneous vagus nerve stimulation has been proposed as an alternative method for the treatment of various psychiatric disorders. The application of this device in refractory seizures is still not conclusive concerning the efficacy, and future trials are needed [70].

### 6.6 Ablative procedure

There are multiple varieties of ablative procedures for refractory seizures, including:

#### *6.6.1 SEEG-guide radiofrequency thermos coagulation*

SEEG-guide RF-TC has been developed and expanded [71]. A single or multiple lesionotomy by coagulation should be performed between continuous electrode contacts, with progressive increasing in power till the impedance suddenly changes indicating that thermos coagulation has occurred. The best response was observed in patients with periventricular heterotopia, results showed pooled seizure free rate of 23% and response rate of 58% [71].

### *6.6.2 Laser interstitial thermal therapy (LITT)*

LITT is also a stereotactic laser ablation (SLA). The laser applicator sheath is placed and lesionotomy performed with precise imaging technique using MRI. The ablation is carried out under continuous monitoring of MRI thermal image near real time. In MTLE, improvement of 58% was achieved according to Engle scale I outcome after 1 year [72].

### *6.6.3 Radiosurgery*

Radiosurgery has been used for (MTLS), gelastic epilepsy associated with hypothalamic hamartomas and epilepsy with vascular malformation, and it has demonstrated a decrease in seizure frequency in MTLS, hamartomas of the hypothalamus, and AVM. Delayed therapeutic effect must be considered in treatment decision [73], and recently, it has been shown that radiosurgery of corpus callosum may in some cases result in seizure reduction [74].

## 7. Current surgical challenges and the future

Despite the advances in technology and surgical technique, control of seizure in the best centers ranges between 15 and 75% and has no changed for the last three decades [75]. Mechanism of epileptogenesis may involve epileptic network rather than a single focus. Using the depth electrodes, independent ictal onset with same semiology from the hippocampus, entorhinal cortex, and amygdala in the same patient with medial temporal lobe epilepsy can be detected. It is known that unidentified epileptogenic source happens in 50% of patients treated surgically [23].

It is known that 10–15 years after surgery, seizure control declines with only 15–50% remaining seizure free [8].

In cases of more than one pathology, such as MTLS, migratory disorder, or tumor, seizure is usually not controlled unless sources resection is addressed [76].

Neuropsychological tests demonstrated cognitive deficit in most patients without tumors or cavernomas [77]. Epileptogenic network is partially supported by Microanalysis (elevation of glutamate levels in epileptogenic region and greater increase after ictal onset, 7 T-MR spectroscopy detecting the mitochondrial function in cortico-subcortical area) and electrophysiological connectivity [24].

Open-loop device for constant stimulation of the anterior thalami (not approved by FDA) could control the epileptogenic site and the lesional area, reducing the seizure in less than 50% of patients in a clinical trial [78].

For better understanding of the epileptogenic network, we need bioelectric integrated telemetered intracranial monitoring. The next advances will need a molecular biosensor with wireless transmission of critical data. Medicine and surgery are not able to control seizure in all epileptic patients yet.

The new surgical roadmap comprises enhancing research, through collaboration, bioinformatics, information scientist biomedical informatics, and information technology.

## 8. Conclusions

Despite the recent advances in the technical aspects of surgical treatment and the diagnostic approaches in PR patients, outcome concerning seizure freedom remains within the same range as during the last decades. Resective and disconnecting surgery may have reached the ceiling of their possibilities, and alternative additional procedures are needed to achieve better outcome. Scientific knowledge about the epileptogenic zone is still evolving and will be the main key for the treatment of PR patients and seizure outcome.

Prospective multicentric studies are needed for the application of new diagnostic procedures, surgical techniques, including the minimally invasive ones and response neurostimulator for the state-of-the art epilepsy surgery.


## Author details

Ahmad Tamimi[1*], Malik Juweid[2] and Iskandar Tamimi[3]

1 Faculty of Medicine, Department of Neurosurgery, University of Jordan, Amman, Jordan

2 Faculty of Medicine, Department of Radiology and Nuclear Medicine, University of Jordan Hospital, Amman, Jordan

3 Faculty of Medicine, Department of Orthopedic Surgery, Carlos Haya Regional University Hospital, University of Malaga, Malaga, Spain

*Address all correspondence to: aftamimi@hotmail.com

## References

[1] Kobau R, Zahran H, Thurman DJ, Zack MM, Henry TR, Schachter SC, et al. Epilepsy surveillance among adults--19 states, behavioral risk factor surveillance system, 2005. MMWR Surveillance Summaries. 2008;**57**(6):1-20

[2] Zack MM, Kobau R. National and state estimates of the numbers of adults and children with active epilepsy - United States, 2015. MMWR. Morbidity and Mortality Weekly Report. 2017;**66**(31):821-825

[3] GBD. 2015 neurological disorders collaborator group. Global, regional, and national burden of neurological disorders during 1990-2015: A systematic analysis for the global burden of disease study 2015. Lancet Neurology. 2017;**16**(11):877-897

[4] DeGiorgio CM, Curtis A, Carapetian A, Hovsepian D, Krishnadasan A, Markovic D. Why are epilepsy mortality rates rising in the United States? A population-based multiple cause-of-death study. BMJ Open. 2020;**10**(8):e035767

[5] Vossler DG, Brian H. Kopell, Epilepsy surgery for complications, Epilepsy Surgery Updated: 11 Dec ,2018

[6] Vakharia VN, Duncan JS, Witt JA, Elger CE, Staba R, Engel J. Getting the best outcomes from epilepsy surgery. Annals of Neurology. 2018;**83**(4):676-690

[7] Jobst BC. Consensus over individualism: Validation of the ILAE definition for drug resistant epilepsy. Epilepsy Currents. 2015;**15**(4):172-173

[8] Kwan P, Arzimanoglou A, Berg AT, Brodie MJ, Allen Hauser W, Mathern G, et al. Definition of drug resistant epilepsy: Consensus proposal by the ad hoc task force of the ILAE commission on therapeutic strategies. Epilepsia. 2010;**51**(6):1069-1077

[9] Malmgren K, Sullivan M, Ekstedt G, Kullberg G, Kumlien E. Health-related quality of life after epilepsy surgery: A Swedish multicenter study. Epilepsia. 1997;**38**(7):830-838

[10] Engel J. Why is there still doubt to cut it out? Epilepsy Currents. 2013;**13**(5):198-204

[11] Poon TL. Presurgical evaluation of epilepsy surgery. In: Misciagnas S, editor. Epilepsy-Update on Classification, Etiologies, Instrumental Diagnosis, and Treatment. Chapter 13. London, UK: IntechOpen; 2021. pp. 1-18

[12] Begley CE, Famulari M, Annegers JF, Lairson DR, Reynolds TF, Coan S, et al. The cost of epilepsy in the United States: An estimate from population-based clinical and survey data. Epilepsia. 2000;**41**(3):342-351

[13] Berg AT. Efficacy of epilepsy surgery: What are the questions today? Nature Reviews. Neurology. 2011;**7**(6):311-312

[14] Téllez-Zenteno JF, Dhar R, Wiebe S. Long-term seizure outcomes following epilepsy surgery: A systematic review and meta-analysis. Brain. 2005;**128**(Pt 5): 1188-1198

[15] Epilepsy Centers [Internet]. Epilepsy Foundation. Available from: https://www.epilepsy.com/treatment/epilepsy-centers. [Accessed: July 25, 2022]

[16] Berg AT, Langfitt J, Shinnar S, Vickrey BG, Sperling MR, Walczak T,

et al. How long does it take for partial epilepsy to become intractable? Neurology. 2003;**60**(2):186-190

[17] Jehi L. The epileptogenic zone: Concept and definition. Epilepsy Currents. 2018;**18**(1):12-16

[18] Nowell M, Miserocchi A, McEvoy AW, Duncan JS. Advances in epilepsy surgery. Journal of Neurology, Neurosurgery, and Psychiatry. 2014;**85**(11):1273-1279

[19] David O, Blauwblomme T, Job AS, Chabardès S, Hoffmann D, Minotti L, et al. Imaging the seizure onset zone with stereo-electroencephalography. Brain. 2011;**134**(10):2898-2911

[20] Wennberg R, Ladino LD, Téllez-Zenteno JF. On the renaissance of stereotactic EEG and its interpretation. Canadian Journal of Neurological Sciences. 2018;**45**(3):255-258

[21] McIntosh AM, Averill CA, Kalnins RM, Mitchell LA, Fabinyi GCA, Jackson GD, et al. Long-term seizure outcome and risk factors for recurrence after extratemporal epilepsy surgery. Epilepsia. 2012;**53**(6):970-978

[22] Cavus I, Kasoff WS, Cassaday MP, Jacob R, Gueorguieva R, Sherwin RS, et al. Extracellular metabolites in the cortex and hippocampus of epileptic patients. Annals of Neurology. 2005;**57**(2):226-235

[23] Pan JW, Kim JH, Cohen-Gadol A, Pan C, Spencer DD, Hetherington HP. Regional energetic dysfunction in hippocampal epilepsy. Acta Neurologica Scandinavica. 2005;**111**(4):218-224

[24] Anyanwu C, Motamedi GK. Diagnosis and surgical treatment of drug-resistant epilepsy. Brain Sciences. 2018;**8**(4):49

[25] Duncan JS. Selecting patients for epilepsy surgery: Synthesis of data. Epilepsy & Behavior. 2011;**20**(2):230-232

[26] Cascino GD, Brinkmann BH. Advances in the surgical Management of Epilepsy: Drug-resistant focal epilepsy in the adult patient. Neurologic Clinics. 2021;**39**(1):181-196

[27] Baxendale S, Thompson P. Beyond localization: The role of traditional neuropsychological tests in an age of imaging. Epilepsia. 2010;**51**(11):2225-2230

[28] Baxendale S. Reply to comment on indications and expecttions for neuropdychological assessment in epilepsy surgery in children and adults. Epileptic Disorders. 2019;**21**:612-613

[29] Cascino GD, Trenerry MR, So EL, Sharbrough FW, Shin C, Lagerlund TD, et al. Routine EEG and temporal lobe epilepsy: Relation to long-term EEG monitoring, quantitative MRI, and operative outcome. Epilepsia. 1996;**37**(7):651-656

[30] Pataraia E, Lurger S, Serles W, Lindinger G, Aull S, Leutmezer F, et al. Ictal scalp EEG in unilateral mesial temporal lobe epilepsy. Epilepsia. 1998;**39**(6):608-614

[31] Schulz R, Lüders HO, Hoppe M, Tuxhorn I, May T, Ebner A. Interictal EEG and ictal scalp EEG propagation are highly predictive of surgical outcome in mesial temporal lobe epilepsy. Epilepsia. 2000;**41**(5):564-570

[32] Rodionov R, Vollmar C, Nowell M, Miserocchi A, Wehner T, Micallef C, et al. Feasibility of multimodal 3D neuroimaging to guide implantation of intracranial EEG electrodes. Epilepsy Research. 2013;**107**(1):91-100

[33] Bulacio JC, Chauvel P, McGonigal A. Stereoelectroencephalography: Interpretation. Journal of Clinical Neurophysiology. 2016;**33**(6):503-510

[34] Cossu M, Chabardès S, Hoffmann D, Lo RG. Presurgical evaluation of intractable epilepsy using stereo-electro-encephalography methodology: Principles, technique and morbidity. Neuro-Chirurgie. 2008;**54**(3):367-373

[35] Focke NK, Bonelli SB, Yogarajah M, Scott C, Symms MR, Duncan JS. Automated normalized FLAIR imaging in MRI-negative patients with refractory focal epilepsy. Epilepsia. 2009;**50**(6):1484-1490

[36] Zijlmans M, Huiskamp G, Hersevoort M, Seppenwoolde JH, van Huffelen AC, Leijten FSS. EEG-fMRI in the preoperative work-up for epilepsy surgery. Brain. 2007;**130**(Pt 9):2343-2353

[37] Loring DW, Meador KJ, Westerveld M. The Wada test in the evaluation for epilepsy surgery. Neurosciences Journal. 2000;**5**(4):203-208

[38] Vivekanada U. Redefining the role of Magnwtowncephalograph in refractory seizure. European Journal of epilepsy. 2020;**83**:70-75

[39] Borna A, Carter TR, Colombo AP, Jau YY, McKay J, Weisend M, et al. Non-invasive functional-brain-imaging with an OPM-based magnetoencephalography system. PLoS One. 2020;**15**(1):e0227684

[40] Mendes Coelho VC, Morita ME, Amorim BJ, Ramos CD, Yasuda CL, Tedeschi H, et al. Automated online quantification method for 18F-FDG positron emission tomography/CT improves detection of the epileptogenic zone in patients with Pharmacoresistant epilepsy. Frontiers in Neurology. 2017;**8**:453

[41] Ponisio MR, Zempel JM, Day BK, Eisenman LN, Miller-Thomas MM, Smyth MD, et al. The role of SPECT and PET in Epillepsy. AJR. American Journal of Roentgenology. 2021;**216**(3):759-768

[42] Shin HW, Jewells V, Sheikh AJ, Zhu H, An H, Wei Gao W, et al. Initial experience in hybrid PET-MRI for evaluation of refractory focal onset epilepsy. Seizure. 2015;**31**:1-4

[43] Juhász C, Asano E, Shah A, Chugani DC, Batista CE, Muzik O, et al. Focal decreases of cortical $GABA_A$ receptor binding remote from the primary seizure focus: What do they indicate? Epilepsia. 2009;**50**(2):240-250

[44] Kumar A, Asano E, Chugani HT. α-[$^{11}$C]-methyl-L-tryptophan PET for tracer localization of epileptogenic brain regions: Clinical studies. Biomarkers in Medicine. 2011;**5**(5):577-584. DOI: 10.2217/bmm.11.68

[45] Engel JJ. What can we do for people with drug-resistant epilepsy? The 2016 Wartenberg lecture. Neurology. 2016;**87**:2483-2489

[46] Sperling MR, Barshow S, Nei M, Asadi-Pooya AA. A reappraisalof mortality after epilepsy surgery. Neurology. 2016;**86**:1938-1944

[47] Soriano SG, McManus ML. Anestetic and postoperative ICU care. In: Cataletepe O, Gallo JL, editors. Pediatric Epilepsy Surgery. Thieme, New York: Stuttgart; 2010. pp. 113-118

[48] Maesawa S, Nakatsubo D, Fujii M, Iijima K, Kato S, Ishizaki T, et al. Application of awake surgery for epilepsy in clinical practice. Neurologia Medico-Chirurgica (Tokyo). 2018;**58**(10):442-452

[49] Dubeau F, McLachlan RS. Invasive electrographic recording techniques in temporal lobe epilepsy can. Journal of the Neurological Sciences. 2000;**27**(Suppl. 1):S29-S34. discussion S50-2

[50] Sperling MR. Clinical challenges in invasive monitoring in epilepsy surgery. Epilepsia. 1997;**38**(suppl. 4):s6-s12

[51] Adelson PD, O'Rourke DK, Albright AL. Chronic invasive monitoring for identifying seizure foci in children. Neurosurgery Clinics of North America. 1995;**6**(3):491-504

[52] Chakraborty A, Rutka J. Surgical approaches to epilepsy. Therapy. 2010;**7**(5):467-479

[53] Cataltepe O, Jallo GI. Surgical management of lesional temporal lobe epilepsy. In: Pediatric Epilepsy Surgery-Assessment and Surgical Treatment. New York, Stuttgart: Thieme; 2011. pp. 161-173

[54] Benifla M, Otsubo H, Ochi A, et al. Temporal lobe surgery for intractable epilepsy in children: An analysis of outcomes in 126 children. Neurosurgery. 2006;**59**(6):1203-1213

[55] Larkin CM, O'Brien DF, Maheshwari D. Anaesthesia for epilepsy surgery. BJA Education. 2019;**19**(12):383-e389

[56] Wiebe S, Warren B, Girvin T, John P. Eliasziw, M, a randomized, controlled trial of surgery for temporal-lobe epilepsy. New England Journal of Medicine. 2001;**345**(5):311-3182

[57] Schramm J. Temporal lobe epilepsy surgery and the quest for optimal extent of resection: A review. Epilepsia. 2008;**49**(8):1296-1307

[58] Bonini F, McGonigal A, Scavarda D, et al. Predictive factors of surgical outcome in frontal lobe epilepsy explored with stereoelectroencephalography. Neurosurgery. 2018;**83**(2):217-225

[59] Englot DJ, Wang DD, Rolston JD, et al. Rates and predictors of long-term seizure freedom after frontal lobe epilepsy surgery: A systematicreview and meta-analysis. Journal of Neurosurgery. 2012;**116**:1042-1048

[60] Laoprasert P, Ojemann JG, Handler MH. Insular epilepsy surgery. Epilepsia. 2017;**58**(suppl. 1):35-45

[61] Asadollahi M, Sperling MR, Rabiei AH, Asadi-Pooya AA. Drug-resistant parietal lobe epilepsy: Clinical manifestations and surgeryoutcome. Epileptic Disorders. 2017;**19**:35-39

[62] Luat AF, Asano E, Kumar A, Chugani H, Sood S. Corpus callosotomy for intractable epilepsy revisited: The Children's Hospital of Michigan series. Journal of Child Neurology. 2017;**32**(7):624-629

[63] Graham D, Tisdall MM, Gill D. Corpus callosotomy outcomes in pediatric patients: A systematic review. Epilepsia. 2016;**57**(7):1053-1068

[64] Smyth MD, Vellimana AK, Asano E, Sood S. Corpus callosotomy—Open and endoscopic surgical techniques. Epilepsia. 2017;**58**(Suppl. 1):73-79

[65] Werhahn KJ, Landvogt C, Klimpe S, Buchholz HG, Yakushev I, Siessmeier T, et al. Decreased dopamine D2/D3-receptor binding in temporal lobe epilepsy: An [18F] Fallypride PET study. Epilepsia. 2006;**47**(8):1392-1396

[66] Morrell MJ. RNS system in epilepsy study group. Responsive cortical

stimulation of the treatment of medically intractable partial epilepsy. Neurology. 2011;77:1295-1304

[67] Nair D, Laxer KL, Weber PB, Murro AM, Park YD, Barkely GL, et al. Nine year prospective efficacy and safety of brain responsive neurostimulator for focal epilepsy. Neurology. 2020;**95**:e1244-e1256

[68] Salanova V. Deep brain stimulation for epilepsy. Epilepsy & Behavior. 2018;**88s**:21-24

[69] Benbadis SR, Geler E, Ryvlin P, Schachter S, Wheless J, Doyle W, Vale FL. Putting in all togother: Options for intractable epilepsy: An uptodate alogarithm on the use of epilepsy surgery and neuro stimulation. Epilepsy & Behavior. 2018;**88S**:33-38

[70] Lampros M, Vlachos N, Zigouris A, Voulgaris S, Alexious GA. Transcutaneous Vagus nerve stimulation(t-VNsS) and epilepsy: A systematic review of literature. Seizure. 2021;**91**:40-48

[71] Bourdillon P, Cucherat M, Isnard J, Ostrowsky-Coste K, Catenoix H, Guenot M, et al. Stereo-electroencephalography-guided radiofrequency thermocoagulation in patients with focal epilepsy: A systematic review and meta-analysis. Epilepsia. 2018;**59**(12):2296-2304

[72] Wu C, Jermakowicz WJ, Chakravorti S, Cajigas I, Sharan AD, Jagid JR, et al. Effects of surgical targeting in laser interdtitial thermal therapy for mesial temporal sclerosis: A multicenter study of 234 patients. Epilepsia. 2019;**60**(6):1171-1183

[73] McGonigal A, Sahgal A, De Salles A, Hayashi M, Levivier M, Ma L, et al. Radiosurgery for epilepsy; systematic review and international s\stereotactic radiosurgery society. Epilepsy Research. 2017;**137**:123-131

[74] Markosian C, Patel S, Kosach S, Goodman RR, Tomycz LD. Corpus callostomy in the modern era; origins, efficacy, technical variation, complications and indications. World Neurosrug. 2022;**159**:146-155

[75] Bulacio JC, Wong C, Gonzalez-Martinez J, Kotagal P, Nair D, Najm I, et al. Long-term seizure outcome after respective surgery in patients evaluated with intracranial electrodes. Epilepsia. 2012;**53**(10):1722-1730

[76] Vale FL, Vivas AC, Manwaring J, Schoenberg MR, Benbadis SR. Temporal lobe epilepsy and cavernous malformation; surgical strategies and long-term outcomes. Act. Neurochin(Wein). 2015;**157**:1887-1895

[77] Privitera M. Epilepsy treatment: A futurist view. Epilepsy Current. 2017;**17**(4):204-2013

[78] Dalkilic CB. Neurostimulation device used in treatment of epilepsy. Current Treatment Options in Neurology. 2017;**19**(2):7

Chapter 6

# Transcranial Magnetic Stimulation, Connectome and Its Clinical Applications

*Ming-Him Yuen*


## Abstract

Transcranial magnetic stimulation is an non-invasive method of neuromodulation. It uses magnetic field to induce generation of current for cortical stimulation. It can modulate the altered equilibrium in cortical excitability by magnetic field. Though it is famous for its application in treating psychiatric diseases, it has many other applications. Since its introduction in 1985, it has been used to check the integrity of motor pathway. With more understanding of the technique, it has been started to be used to check the integrity of other brain connections like speech and vision. Due to its ability of neuromodulation, it has also been used in cortical mapping in neurosurgery and neurological function rehabilitation.


**Keywords:** transcranial magnetic stimulation, TMS, neuromodulation, neurorehabilitation, cortical mapping

## 1. Introduction

Transcranial magnetic stimulation, which is commonly abbreviated as TMS, is an non-invasive method of cortical stimulation by the use of electromagnetic field. It is a safe and effective method of neuromodulation. It has been used as a tool for checking the integrity of neuronal pathway for prognosis estimation after insult. It is an FDA approved treatment for several psychiatric diseases. It is now also used for rehabilitation of different neurological deficits, like motor rehabilitation and dysphasia. Its neuromodulation property is used in treating Parkinson's disease and epilepsy. With the advancement in navigated TMS, it has been applied in cortical mapping, especially in neurosurgical operative planning.

## 2. History

The foundation of TMS is inspired by the ideas of Luigi Galvani, an Italian doctor, and Michael Faraday, a British physicist. The former first experimented the electrical stimulation of muscles and nerve fibers in the late eighteenth century while the latter in 1831 discovered that the relationship of electrical energy and magnetic field was reciprocal [1, 2]. Based on their theories, researchers had tried to study the effects of electromagnetic stimulation of brain, but most attempts were in vane due to technical limitations [3]. It was not until 1985 when Anthony Barker, a British engineer from the University of Sheffield, presented to the world about his invention of the first practical electromagnetic stimulation device for human use and his successful demonstration of the influence of electromagnetic stimulation on motor cortex of the human brain [4]. He and his associates placed a single Faraday coil to the scalp above the left cerebral motor strip of the subject to induce movement in the right hand. The outfit of the device was showed in **Figure 1** [4]. Though this machine was slow in charging and the elevation of temperature of the coil limited its repetitive uses, it marked the start of modern TMS era.

Based on his inventions, researches were done to expand clinical applications of TMS. In 1995, the first pilot clinical trial was published reporting the results of TMS in treatment of depression [5]. In 2002, Canadian Association of Health approved the medical results and benefits of repetitive TMS (rTMS) [6]. The first The United States Food and Drug Administration (FDA) approval of TMS was given in 2008 in treatment of depression [3]. In 2009, FDA also approved TMS for cortical mapping. Since late 1990s, applications of TMS on neurological rehabilitation and treatment of different neurological diseases have been the focus of researches. TMS on motor rehabilitation and dysphasia is gaining more and more support from evidences in literature [7–10]. With advancement in technology, introduction of navigated TMS provides more precise application of TMS in mapping and treatment.

## 3. Equipment

There are several companies producing TMS-related equipment. The basic requirements of TMS service include a transcranial magnetic stimulator and coils. The examples of stimulators and coils are shown in **Figures 2** and **3** [11, 12]. Circular coils are the basic type of coils. Figure-of-eight coils, or also known as butterfly coils, consist of two sets of coils arranged in a figure-of-eight fashion to make the strength of the magnetic field generated more focused when compared with traditional circular coils [13]. They are commonly used for treatment. **Figure 4** shows the magnetic field strength induced by circular coil and figure-of-eight coil, respectively. Double-cone coil has two large cup-shaped windings positioned side by side. It is used

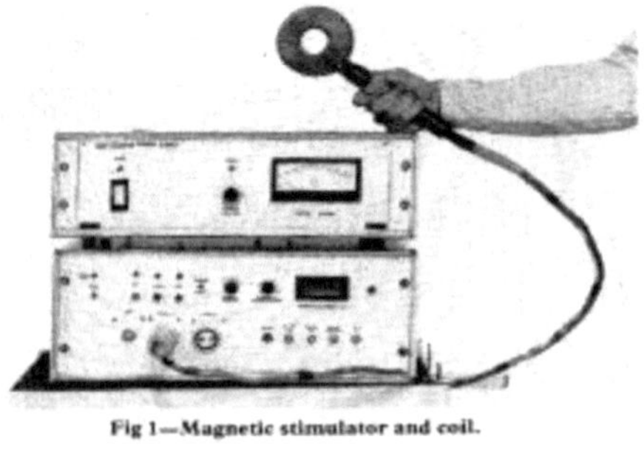


**Figure 1.**
*TMS machine invented by Dr. Anthony Barker [4].*

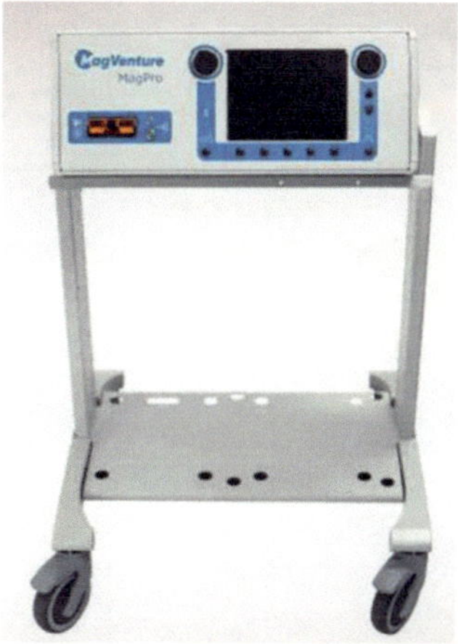

**Figure 2.**
*Example of a transcranial magnetic stimulator [11].*

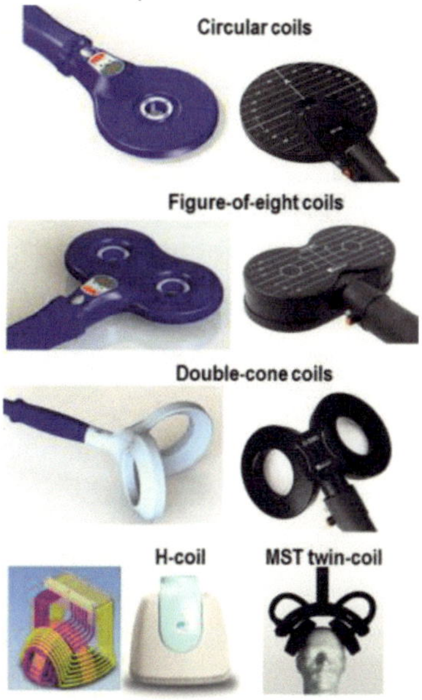


**Figure 3.**
*Different types of commonly used coils [12].*

to stimulate deep-seated structure. H-coil is a special designed coil that is also used to stimulate deep seated target. Apart from the appearance of the coils, treatment coils may also be equipped with specific cooling system for heat dissipation. Heat dissipation is particularly important in more aggressive treatment protocol like theta burst stimulation (TBS) protocol. Liquid cooling system and forced-air cooling system are the commonest cooling systems employed.

Some adjuncts can be used during TMS. Devices recording motor-evoked potential and electroencephalography (EEG) are frequently utilized. For navigated TMS (nTMS), sensor, localizers and software for MRI navigation are essential components on top of the basic requirements.

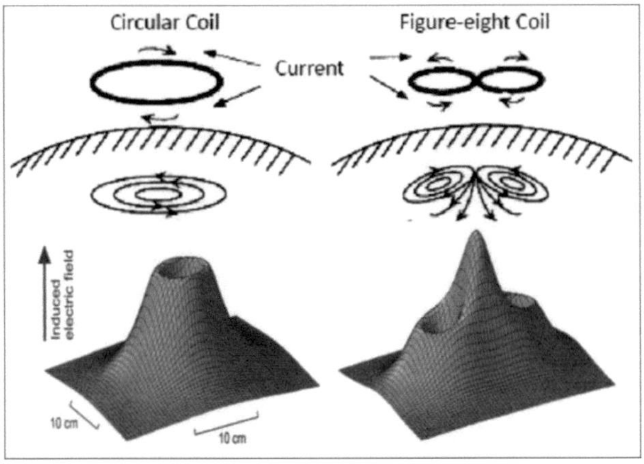


**Figure 4.**
*Magnetic field strength induced by circular coil and figure-of-eight coil, respectively [13].*

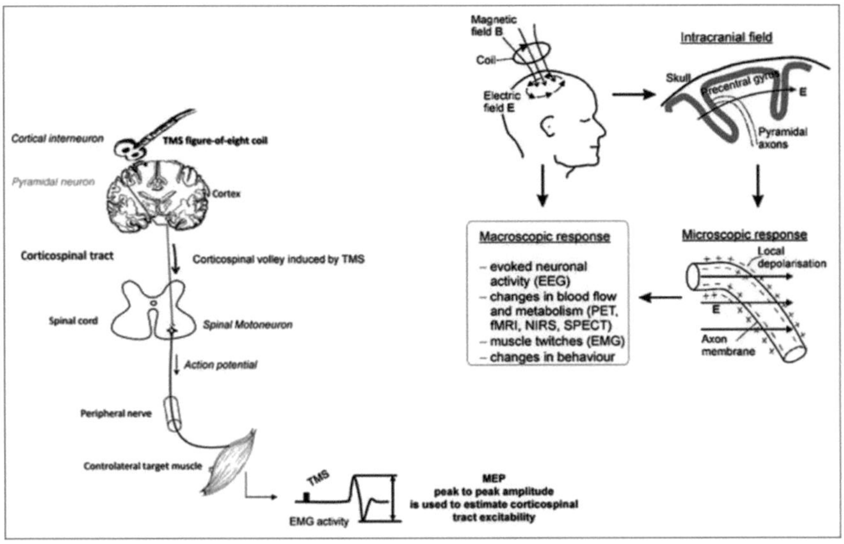


**Figure 5.**
*Mechanism of action for TMS [13].*

## 4. Mechanism of actions and theories

When current flows through the coil, magnetic field is generated by Ampere's law. When the coil is placed over the scalp, the magnetic field strength generated passes through the scalp and skull then affects a nearby neuron. The magnetic field generates current in that particular neuron by Faraday's law to cause depolarization of the neuron and propagation of action potential. If the neuron affected is located in motor cortex, the cascade process induced by TMS triggers a muscle movement which can be recorded by electromyography. This firing of impulse passes through the pathway to the end organ to produce a specific response. If this pathway is not intact, the impulse of action potential cannot reach the end organ, and no response can be produced. **Figure 5** shows how TMS triggers the cascade [13]. The magnetic field strength generated ranged from 1.5 to 3 Tesla [14, 15]. Typical figure-of-eight coil is able to activate cortical neurons 1.5–3 cm beneath the scalp [16].

The method of pulse delivery leads to different neuromodulative outcomes. Single-pulse delivery produces immediate effect without causing any long-lasting effect, i.e., no after effect. This mode of pulse delivery is best used for cortical mapping and checking the integrity of neuronal pathways. Pattern TMS, including repetitive TMS (rTMS) and theta burst stimulation (TBS) pattern, on the other hand produces persistent effect beyond the stimulation period, i.e., it possesses after effect. This property is useful in provision of treatment and rehabilitation. rTMS is the delivery of a number of trains of repetitive stimulation at a fixed frequency. rTMS may have intervals of breaks in between trains of stimulation. rTMS delivered at 1 Hertz (Hz) is considered as low frequency, while rTMS delivered at 5 Hz or above is considered as high frequency. TBS pattern describes the delivery of 3 pulses at 50 Hz in every 200 microseconds. TBS pattern can be given in an intermittent fashion or in a continuous fashion. In the intermittent theta burst stimulation pattern (iTBS), 600 pulses of stimulations are given in 190 seconds in a fashion that a 2-second train of TBS stimulation followed by 8 seconds of break in every 10 seconds. In the continuous theta burst stimulation paradigm (cTBS), 600 pulses of stimulations are given in TBS pattern uninterruptedly for 40 seconds [16]. Neuromodulation makes use of the after effect which can be classified as excitatory or inhibitory. High-frequency rTMS and iTBS are found to have excitatory effects, while, on the contrary, low-frequency rTMS and cTBS are associated with inhibitory effects [16]. **Figure 6** shows the summary of effects of rTMS and TBS [17].

The exact mechanism of how after effect of TMS helps in neuromodulation remains unclear. The most popular theory is interhemispheric balance theory, which is also known as interhemispheric rivalry theory [18, 19]. It is believed that each cerebral hemisphere inhibits its contralateral counterpart via the corpus callosum and the two sides are at a balanced status. When a pathology occurs in one side, this balance is disturbed. The inhibitory effect from the normal contralateral side will be uncounteracted in the lesioned side, leading to symptoms. Therefore, the aim of TMS is to restore the balance, either by inhibiting the normal contralateral side or stimulating the pathological side (**Figure 7**).

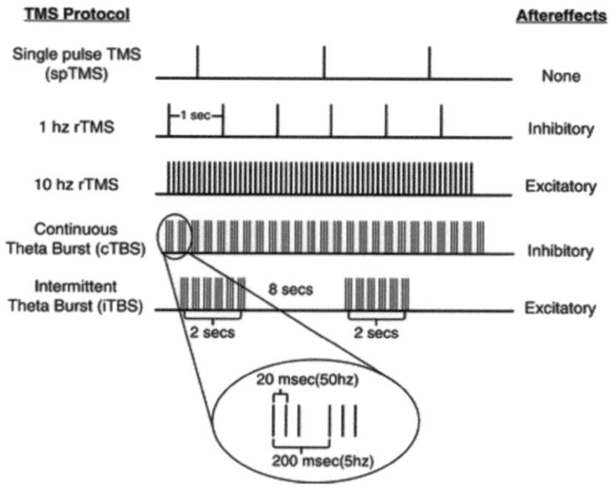


**Figure 6.**
*Summary of effects of rTMS and TBS [17].*

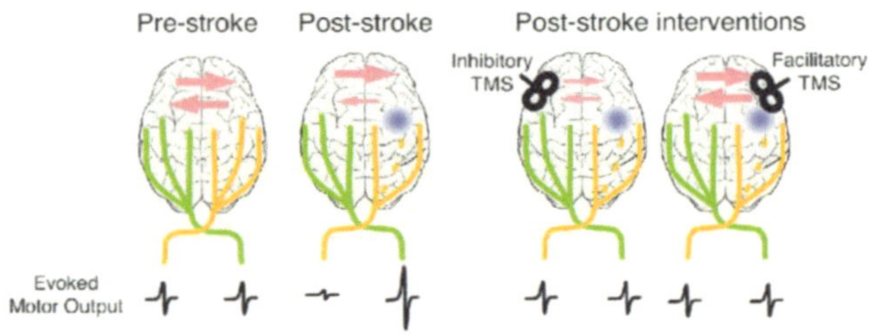


**Figure 7.**
*Interhemispheric rivalry theory [18].*

## 5. Contraindications and risks of TMS

The contraindications are mostly related to the exposure of the magnetic field. The absolute contraindication is the presence of ferromagnetic implant in head and neck region, including tattoo on face. Though TMS can be one of the treatments for convulsion, known history of convulsion or suboptimally controlled convulsion, medications that potentially lower seizure threshold and alcoholism may be the exclusion criteria in some of the TMS centers [20]. Heating issue of metallic implant is another concern in patient selection. Eddy currents induced in conductive surface electrodes and implants can cause them to heat up [20]. The temperature increase depends on the shape, size, orientation, conductivity, and surrounding tissue properties of the electrode or implant as well as the TMS coil type, position, and stimulation parameters. Silver and gold are highly conductive and can produce heat excessively, potentially leading to skin burn or even brain tissue damage. Titanium tends to have low heating profile and is safe for TMS [20]. Although there are successful and uneventful TMS treatment done on pregnant ladies [20], pregnancy is still a concern in many centers. Pediatric safety is yet to be confirmed. A systematic review shows that TMS is apparently safe for pediatric patients aged 6 or above [21]. However, there is currently no enough data to demonstrate safety or hazard for individuals below 6 years of age [21].

Transient hearing impairment, convulsion, syncope, local scalp discomfort, headache and acute psychiatric changes have been reported as TMS-related risks [20]. The incidence for significant complications is low. Therefore, TMS is overall a safe procedure. Summary of potential risks is shown in **Table 1** [20].

## 6. Indications

There are many indications and may be grossly divided into two categories, namely therapeutic and non-therapeutic.

### 6.1 Therapeutic

#### *6.1.1 Depression*

Major depression is the first FDA approved indication for TMS. Multiple meta-analyses suggest that rTMS has a comparable effect to electroconvulsive therapy and antidepressants. It shows significant improvement in both helpless and anhedonic symptoms, with squared deviation from mean (SDM) 1.34 and 1.87, respectively [22]. The standard protocol is to deliver 10 Hz stimulation to left dorsolateral prefrontal cortex over 4–6 week in once-daily stimulation session. Other treatment protocols are also available [22]. iTBS is also proven to be as effective as the standard rTMS protocol with response rate of 36.7% when compared with 33.3% in standard rTMS protocol [23].

#### *6.1.2 Obsessive and compulsive disorders (OCD)*

OCD is another FDA approved indication for TMS. Multiple meta-analyses suggest rTMS is effective [24]. There are a couple of rTMS protocols with different targets like supplementary motor area, orbitofrontal cortex and dorsolateral prefrontal cortex [25, 26]. cTBS may also show a therapeutic effect in treating OCD at 6 weeks in terms of Yale–Brown Obsessive–Compulsive Scale and Hamilton Anxiety Rating Scale [27].

#### *6.1.3 Smoking cessation*

FDA clearance for TMS on smoking cessation was granted in 2020. It was based on a pivotal randomized controlled trial sponsored by a pharmacological company [28]. It used H coil to stimulate lateral prefrontal cortex and insula by facilitatory rTMS and achieved 28.0% continuous quit rate at week 18 compared to 11.7% in sham group [28]. With this landmark paper, more evidence was concluded from systematic reviews and meta-analyses in proving the effectiveness of rTMS on smoking cessation [29].

#### *6.1.4 Schizophrenia*

Stanford et al. suggested that negative symptoms appeared to be associated with hypoactivity of the dorsolateral prefrontal cortex of the brain while positive symptoms, particularly auditory hallucination, appeared to be associated with hyperactivity in the left temporo-parietal cortex [30]. Therefore, high-frequency rTMS at dorsolateral prefrontal cortex was suggested for negative symptoms and low-frequency rTMS at left temporo-parietal cortex for positive symptoms. Meta-analyses show the clinical improvement for the mentioned protocol with p value 0.002 [31, 32]. Goh et al. found that iTBS given to left dorsolateral prefrontal cortex was also effective in treating negative symptoms of schizophrenia with a p value of 0.004 [33].

#### *6.1.5 Migraine with aura*

Migraine with aura is another FDA approved indication which was announced in 2017. There are different protocols involving facilitatory stimulation over left dorsolateral prefrontal cortex or left motor cortex [34]. A meta-analysis shows effectiveness of TMS in treating migraine with aura [34]. Prophylactic inhibitory rTMS at vertex in patients with known migraine regardless of the presence of aura apparently also reduces migraine median frequency by 12 days per month and median intensity by 6 points [35].

#### *6.1.6 Motor rehabilitation*

Motor deficits after cranial or spinal insults are common. Stroke is one of the major causes. There is no standardized protocol. Inhibitory rTMS or cTBS over motor cortex of the non-lesional side and facilitatory rTMS or iTBS over motor cortex of lesional side are the common choices. Systematic reviews and meta-analyses show that rTMS

| Side effect | Single-pulse TMS | Paired-pulse TMS | Low-frequency rTMS | High-frequency rTMS | Theta burst |
|---|---|---|---|---|---|
| Seizure induction | Rare | Not reported | Rare (usually protective effect) | Possible (1.4% crude risk estimate in epileptic patients; less than 1% in normals) | Possible (one seizure in a normal subject during cTBS) (see para 3.3.3) |
| Transient acute hypomania induction | No | No | Rare | Possible following left prefrontal stimulation | Not reported |
| Syncope | Possible as epiphenomenon (i.e., not related to direct brain effect) | | | Possible | |
| Transient headache, local pain, neck pain, toothache and paresthesia | Possible | Likely possible, but not reported/ addressed | Frequent (see para. 3.3) | Frequent (see para. 3.3) | Possible |
| Transient hearing changes | Possible | Likely possible, but not reported | Possible | Possible | Not reported |
| Transient cognitive/ neuropsychological changes | Not reported | No reported | Overall negligible (see Section 4.6) | Overall negligible (see Section 4.6) | Transient impairment of working memory |
| Burns from scalp electrodes | No | No | Not reported | Occasionally reported | Not reported, but likely possible |
| Induced currents in electrical circuits | Theoretically possible, but described malfunction only if TMS is delivered in close proximity with the electric device (pace-makers, brain stimulators, pumps, intracardiac lines and cochlear implants) | | | | |
| Structural brain changes | Not reported | Not reported | Inconsistent | Inconsistent | Not reported |

| Side effect | Single-pulse TMS | Paired-pulse TMS | Low-frequency rTMS | High-frequency rTMS | Theta burst |
|---|---|---|---|---|---|
| Histoxicity | No | No | Inconsistent | Inconsistent | Not reported |
| Other biological transient effects | Not reported | Not reported | Not reported | Transient hormone (TSH), and blood lactate levels change | Not reported |

**Table 1.**
*Summary of potential side effects of TMS.*

and TBS are effective in improvement of motor function after insult of the brain with 95% confidence interval 0.24–9.71 for upper limb Fugl Meyer assessment [36–38].

Spinal insults, including trauma and post tumor excision, can also lead to motor deficits. Although there are no insults in brain, the corticospinal tract is affected by the spinal insult. A lot of studies support the use of TMS (rTMS or iTBS) in spinal insult patients, particularly incomplete spinal injury cases, and one of the studies shows improvement in lower limb motor score of 5 points with p value 0.004 compared to 1 point in sham group [39–43].

#### *6.1.7 Parkinson's disease*

Parkinson's disease is a relative common but disabling disease. Neuromodulation is one of the treatment approaches. Unlike deep brain stimulation, TMS provides a method of neuromodulation without the need of incision and anesthesia. Currently there are no consensus for the protocol TMS in managing Parkinson's disease. There are different protocols available. Apparently motor symptoms of Parkinson's disease improve after TMS [44–47]. The Movement Disorder Society-Sponsored Revision of the Unified Parkinson's Disease Rating Scale shows 6 points of improvement in Part III at 4 week post-treatment with p value 0.04 [45].

#### *6.1.8 Other therapeutic uses*

rTMS has been reported to be effective in improving nominal aphasia since 2005 [10]. It shows improvement by two standard deviations in Boston Diagnostic Aphasia Examination [10]. Since then, multiple trials have been conducted to test for the efficacy of rTMS on dysphasia. A recent systematic review confirmed that rTMS is an effective tool in post-stroke aphasia rehabilitation [9].

Tinnitus is one of disabling diseases that may not have any effective medical treatment. rTMS was found to be able to reduce the severity of tinnitus [48–50]. Over 16 points of improvement in Tinnitus handicap inventory scores at 6 months post-treatment was observed [49].

Spasticity is common after cerebral insults like stroke. A recent systematic review shows that TMS helps to improve Modified Ashworth Scale of the patients by 0.58 with p value $<0.01$ [51].

Neuropathic pain is one of the big topics in pain management, and TMS is shown to be an effective tool in managing those patients [52, 53].

rTMS is also shown to be effective in rehabilitation of dysphagia after stroke in recent published systematic reviews [54, 55]. The mean difference was −1.03 with p value <0.0001 in Penetration Aspiration Scale after completion of TMS [55].

There are some other fields that researchers and scholars are working on to see if TMS helps in the management. Examples include hemineglect, visual field impairment and epilepsy [56–58].

### 6.2 Non-therapeutic

#### *6.2.1 Diagnostic and prognostic tool*

Single-pulse TMS has been used to stimulate motor cortex to produce motor response since its first introduction in 1985 [1]. With the successful production of motor response, it proves the integrity of motor pathway, from neurons in motor cortex via corticospinal tract to muscle fibers. Disruption in any part along the tract causes failure of motor response production. This property has been used to evaluate the severity of the insult for both diagnosis and estimation of prognosis and to monitor the progress of rehabilitation [59, 60].

#### *6.2.2 Cortical mapping*

FDA first cleared the use of nTMS in cortical mapping in 2009. It can be used for both motor and language mapping. Intraoperative direct cortical stimulation has been the gold standard for cortical mapping. nTMS has been shown to have good accuracy (<10 mm) in motor mapping compared to direct cortical stimulation [61, 62]. The accuracy of nTMS is comparable or even better than functional MRI according to the results from some studies [61]. nTMS has been in used in preoperative planning in neurosurgical operations to maximize the resection of tumors in eloquent areas while preserving neurological functions [63, 64].

## 7. TMS and connectome

Connectome, the concept first introduced by Professor Sporns, is the connection matrix of human brain, which refers to the complete set of structural connections between neurons of the brain [65]. Diseases or cerebral insults cause disruption of the connectome. Diaschesis and vicaration of function, together with homeostatic mechanism of neuroplasticity, help to restore neurological functions which can be demonstrated by TMS in cortical remapping, i.e., detection of shift of stimulation hotspots compared with premorbid state. TMS, at the same time, is also considered as an non-invasive and safe tool to modulate the reconstruction of connectome after insult during the rehabilitation phase [18].

## 8. TMS and EEG

EEG is an non-invasive method of recording brain activity. TMS can produce TMS-related potential and induce different brain oscillation patterns in different parts of the brain [66]. EEG can be used to record TMS-induced activity when TMS stimulated a non-motor function-related circuit. This was first reported by Dr. Cracco in 1989 [67], but it was not in clinical use until recent decades. Concurrent use of TMS and EEG requires the use of specific TMS compatible EEG system due to risks of eddy current generation with traditional EEG electrodes and early saturation of traditional EEG amplifiers by TMS-induced current [68]. Either single pulse, paired pulses or pattern TMS can be used for different assessment purposes [68]. It is often used with functional MRI and navigated TMS to stimulate a specific target or circuit. Researchers have found that changes in TMS-EEG parameters in various psychiatric and neurological diseases [69]. This may lead to future development as a tool for diagnosis and monitor of treatment response [69].

## 9. Our experience in TMS

Our department first introduced TMS service for neuro-rehabilitation for our patients with intracranial or spinal insults in 2018 in outpatient setting (**Figure 8**). To facilitate early inpatient rehabilitation, TMS service was introduced to our in-hospital patients in 2021 as a routine tool of rehabilitation. rTMS and TBS are employed for motor and dysphasia rehabilitation. Despite service cut during COVID-19 period, over 100 cases had received TMS service in our unit. We conducted a prospective pilot trial to compare the 6-month outcome in motor rehabilitation in stroke patients receiving iTBS to stroke patients receiving conventional physiotherapy. There were significant improvement in upper limb Fugl Meyer assessment score and limb power in patients completing ten sessions of iTBS on motor hotspot of the pathological hemisphere.

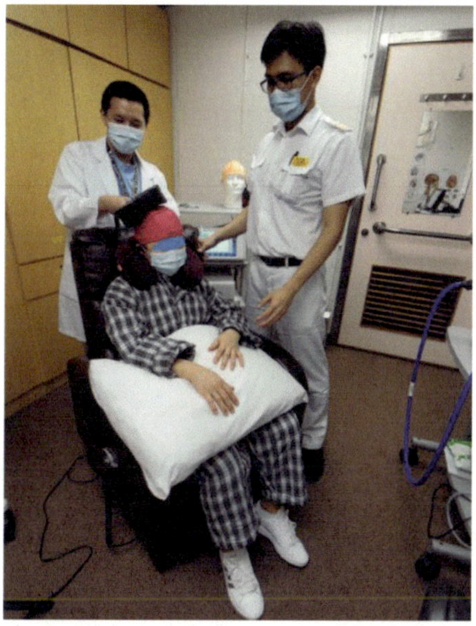

**Figure 8.**
*TMS treatment delivery in outpatient setting.*

## 10. Conclusion

TMS is an non-invasive and safe tool for neuromodulation. It makes use of electromagnetic theory for stimulation of neuronal pathways. It has both diagnostic, prognostic and therapeutic applications. Its applications reflect and demonstrate the connectome inside brain.

## Conflict of interest

The authors declare no conflict of interest.

## Thanks

Special thanks to Dr. Cheung FC[1], Dr. Poon TL[1], Ms. Luk H[2], Mr. Chee B[2], Mr. Au A[3] & colleagues involved in TMS service provision in Queen Elizabeth Hospital, HKSAR

1. Department of Neurosurgery, Queen Elizabeth Hospital, HKSAR.

2. Department of Physiotherapy, Queen Elizabeth Hospital, HKSAR.

3. Department of Speech Therapy, Queen Elizabeth Hospital, HKSAR.

## Author details

Ming-Him Yuen
Department of Neurosurgery, Queen Elizabeth Hospital, Hong Kong SAR, China

*Address all correspondence to: ymh_1985@yahoo.com.hk

## References

[1] Barker A, Freeston I. Transcranial magnetic stimulation. Scholarpedia. 2007;**2**:2936

[2] Reynolds ET. Faraday and the electrical basis of brain activity. Practical Neurology. 2007;**7**(5):331-335

[3] Janicak PG, Dokucu ME. Transcranial magnetic stimulation for the treatment of major depression. Neuropsychiatric Disease and Treatment. 2015;**26**:1549-1560. DOI: 10.2147/NDT.S67477

[4] Barker AT, Jalinous R, Freeston IL. Non-invasive magnetic stimulation of human motor cortex. The Lancet. 1985;**2**:1106-1107

[5] George MS, Wassermann EM, Williams WA, et al. Daily repetitive transcranial magnetic stimulation (rTMS) improves mood in depression. Neuroreport. 1995;**6**(14):1853-1856

[6] Noohi S, Amirsalari S. History, studies and specific uses of repetitive transcranial magnetic stimulation (rTMS) in treating epilepsy. Iranian Journal of Child Neurology. 2016;**10**(1):1-8

[7] Bai Z, Zhang J, Fong KNK. Effects of transcranial magnetic stimulation in modulating cortical excitability in patients with stroke: A systematic review and meta-analysis. Journal of Neuroengineering and Rehabilitation. 2022;**19**:24. DOI: 10.1186/s12984-022-00999-4

[8] Cha T-H, Hwang H-S. Rehabilitation interventions combined with noninvasive brain stimulation on upper limb motor function in stroke patients. Brain Sciences. 2022;**12**(8):994. DOI: 10.3390/brainsci12080994

[9] Arheix-Parras S, Barrios C, Python G, Cogné M, Sibon I, Engelhardt M, et al. A systematic review of repetitive transcranial magnetic stimulation in aphasia rehabilitation: Leads for future studies. Neuroscience and Biobehavioral Reviews. 2021;**127**:212-241. DOI: 10.1016/j.neubiorev.2021.04.008

[10] Naeser MA, Martin PI, Ho M, Treglia E, Kaplan E, Bashir S, et al. Transcranial magnetic stimulation and aphasia rehabilitation. Archives of Physical Medicine and Rehabilitation. 2012;**93**(1 Suppl):S26-S34. DOI: 10.1016/j.apmr.2011.04.026

[11] Magventure TMS therapy. Available from: https://www.magventure.com/us/tms-research/products-overview/research-stimulators/products-6/stimulators-4-2/magpro-x100-4

[12] Lefaucheur JP. Handbook of Clinical Neurology. 2019;**160**:559-580. DOI: 10.1016/B978-0-444-64032-1.00037-0

[13] Udupa K. Transcranial magnetic stimulation in exploring neurophysiology of cortical circuits and potential clinical implications. Indian Journal of Physiology and Pharmacology. 2020;**64**(4):244-257

[14] Walsh V, Pascual-Leone A. Transcranial Magnetic Stimulation: A Neurochronometrics of Mind. Cambridge, Massachusetts: MIT Press; 2003

[15] Turi Z, Normann C, Domschke K, et al. Transcranial magnetic stimulation in psychiatry: Is there a need for electric field standardization? Frontiers in Human Neuroscience. 2021;**15**

[16] Huang YZ, Edwards MJ, Rounis E, Bhatia KP, Rothwell JC. Theta burst stimulation of the human motor cortex. Neuron. 2005;**45**(2):201-206. DOI: 10.1016/j.neuron.2004.12.033

[17] Florida TMS Clinic. Available from: https://www.floridatmsclinic.com/tms-therapy/theta-burst-stimulation

[18] Silasi G, Murphy T. Stroke and the connectome: How connectivity guides therapeutic intervention. Neuron. 2014;**83**:1354-1368. DOI: 10.1016/j.neuron.2014.08.052

[19] Takeuchi N, Oouchida Y, Izumi S. Motor control and neural plasticity through interhemispheric interactions. Neural Plasticity. 2012;**2012**:823285. DOI: 10.1155/2012/823285

[20] Rossi S, Hallett M, Rossini PM, Pascual-Leone A, Safety of TMS Consensus Group. Safety, ethical considerations, and application guidelines for the use of transcranial magnetic stimulation in clinical practice and research. Clinical Neurophysiology. 2009;**120**(12):2008-2039. DOI: 10.1016/j.clinph.2009.08.016

[21] Allen CH, Kluger BM, Buard I. Safety of transcranial magnetic stimulation in children: A systematic review of the literature. Pediatric Neurology. 2017;**68**:3-17. DOI: 10.1016/j.pediatrneurol.2016.12.009

[22] De Risio L, Borgi M, Pettorruso M, et al. Recovering from depression with repetitive transcranial magnetic stimulation (rTMS): A systematic review and meta-analysis of preclinical studies. Translational Psychiatry. 2020;**10**:393. DOI: 10.1038/s41398-020-01055-2

[23] Bulteau S, Laurin A, Pere M, Fayet G, Thomas-Ollivier V, Deschamps T, et al. Intermittent theta burst stimulation (iTBS) versus 10 Hz high-frequency repetitive transcranial magnetic stimulation (rTMS) to alleviate treatment-resistant unipolar depression: A randomized controlled trial (THETA-DEP). Brain Stimulation. 2022;**15**(3):870-880

[24] Paulino T, Pedro S, Ian C, Isa Albuquerque S, Caio Barbosa K, Fernanda G, et al. Transcranial magnetic stimulation for obsessive-compulsive disorder: An updated systematic review and meta-analysis. The Journal of ECT. 2016;**32**(4):262-266

[25] Fitzsimmons SMDD, Van der Werf YD, van Campen AD, Arns M, Sack AT, Hoogendoorn AW, et al. Repetitive transcranial magnetic stimulation for obsessive-compulsive disorder: A systematic review and pairwise/network meta-analysis. Journal of Affective Disorders. 2022;**302**:302-312. DOI: 10.1016/j.jad.2022.01.048

[26] Kammen A, Cavaleri J, Lam J, Frank AC, Mason X, Choi W, et al. Neuromodulation of OCD: A review of invasive and non-invasive methods. Frontiers in Neurology. 2022;**13**:909264. DOI: 10.3389/fneur.2022.909264

[27] Liu W, Shao H, Liao J, Yang D, Ma M, Yang J. Continuous theta-burst stimulation over the right orbitofrontal cortex in treatment-resistant obsessive-compulsive disorder treatment: A randomized sham-controlled trial. International Journal of General Medicine. 2021;**1**:3109-3118. DOI: 10.2147/IJGM.S318069

[28] Zangen A, Moshe H, Martinez D, Barnea-Ygael N, Vapnik T, Bystritsky A, et al. Repetitive transcranial magnetic stimulation for smoking cessation: A pivotal multicenter double-blind randomized controlled trial. World

Psychiatry. 2021;**20**(3):397-404. DOI: 10.1002/wps.20905

[29] Petit B, Dornier A, Meille V, Demina A, Trojak B. Non-invasive brain stimulation for smoking cessation: A systematic review and meta-analysis. Addiction. 2002;**117**(11):2768-2779

[30] Stanford A, Corcoran C, Bulow P, et al. High frequency prefrontal rTMS for the negative symptoms of schizophrenia: A case series. The Journal of ECT. 2011;**27**:11-17

[31] Cole JC, Green Bernacki C, Helmer A, Pinninti N, O'reardon JP. Efficacy of transcranial magnetic stimulation (TMS) in the treatment of schizophrenia: A review of the literature to date. Innovation of Clinical Neuroscience. 2015;**12**(7-8):12-19

[32] Freitas C, Fregni F, Pascual-Leone A. Meta-analysis of the effects of repetitive transcranial magnetic stimulation (rTMS) on negative and positive symptoms in schizophrenia. Schizophrenia Research. 2009;**108**:11-24

[33] Goh KK, Chen CH, Wu TH, Chiu YH, Lu ML. Efficacy and safety of intermittent theta-burst stimulation in patients with schizophrenia: A meta-analysis of randomized sham-controlled trials. Frontiers in Pharmacology. 2022. DOI: 10.3389/fphar.2022.944437

[34] Lan L, Zhang X, Li X, Rong X, Peng Y. The efficacy of transcranial magnetic stimulation on migraine: A meta-analysis of randomized controlled trails. The Journal of Headache and Pain. 2017;**18**(1):86. DOI: 10.1186/s10194-017-0792-4

[35] Hammad AB, Elsharawy RE, Azim GSA. Repetitive transcranial magnetic stimulation as a prophylactic treatment in migraine. The Egyptian Journal of Neurology, Psychiatry and Neurosurgery. 2021;**57**:5. DOI: 10.1186/s41983-020-00254-4

[36] Dionísio A, Duarte IC, Patrício M, Castelo-Branco M. The use of repetitive transcranial magnetic stimulation for stroke rehabilitation: A systematic review. Journal of Stroke and Cerebrovascular Diseases. 2018;**27**(1):1-31. DOI: 10.1016/j.jstrokecerebrovasdis.2017.09.008

[37] Xue T, Yan Z, Meng J, Wang W, Chen S, Wu X, et al. Efficacy of neurostimulations for upper extremity function recovery after stroke: A systematic review and network meta-analysis. Journal of Clinical Medicine. 2022;**11**(20):6162. DOI: 10.3390/jcm11206162

[38] Meehan S, Dao E, Linsdell M, Boyd L. Continuous theta burst stimulation over the contralesional sensory and motor cortex enhances motor learning post-stroke. Neuroscience Letters. 2011;**500**:26-30

[39] Benito J, Kumru H, Murillo N, Costa U, Medina J, Tormo J, et al. Motor and gait improvement in patients with incomplete spinal cord injury induced by high-frequency repetitive transcranial magnetic stimulation. Topics in Spinal Cord Injury Rehabilitation. 2012;**18**(2):106-112

[40] Fassett HJ, Turco CV, El-Sayes J, Lulic T, Baker S, Richardson B, et al. Transcranial magnetic stimulation with intermittent theta burst stimulation alters corticospinal output in patients with chronic incomplete spinal cord injury. Frontiers in Neurology. 2017;**8**. DOI: 10.3389/fneur.2017.00380

[41] Wincek A, Huber J, Leszczyńska K, Fortuna W, Okurowski S, Chmielak K, et al. The long-term effect of treatment

using the transcranial magnetic stimulation rTMS in patients after incomplete cervical or thoracic spinal cord injury. Journal of Clinical Medicine. 2021;**10**(13):2975. DOI: 10.3390/jcm10132975

[42] Leszczyńska K, Wincek A, Fortuna W, Huber J, Łukaszek J, Okurowski S, et al. Treatment of patients with cervical and upper thoracic incomplete spinal cord injury using repetitive transcranial magnetic stimulation. The International Journal of Artificial Organs. 2020;**43**(5):323-331. DOI: 10.1177/0391398819887754

[43] Mittal N, Majdic BC, Peterson CL. Intermittent theta burst stimulation modulates biceps brachii corticomotor excitability in individuals with tetraplegia. Journal of Neuroengineering and Rehabilitation. 2022;**19**(1):73. DOI: 10.1186/s12984-022-01049-9

[44] Wu Y, Cao XB, Zeng WQ, Zhai H, Zhang XQ, Yang XM, et al. Transcranial magnetic stimulation alleviates levodopa-induced dyskinesia in Parkinson's disease and the related mechanisms: A mini-review. Frontiers in Neurology. 2021;**12**:758345. DOI: 10.3389/fneur.2021.758345

[45] Mi TM, Garg S, Ba F, Liu AP, Liang PP, Gao LL, et al. Repetitive transcranial magnetic stimulation improves Parkinson's freezing of gait via normalizing brain connectivity. NPJ Parkinsons Disease. 2020;**6**:16. DOI: 10.1038/s41531-020-0118-0

[46] Khedr EM, Rothwell JC, Shawky OA, Ahmed MA, Hamdy A. Effect of daily repetitive transcranial magnetic stimulation on motor performance in Parkinson's disease. Movement Disorders. 2006;**21**(12):2201-2205. DOI: 10.1002/mds.21089

[47] Brys M, Fox MD, Agarwal S, Biagioni M, Dacpano G, Kumar P, et al. Multifocal repetitive TMS for motor and mood symptoms of Parkinson disease: A randomized trial. Neurology. 2016;**87**(18):1907-1915. DOI: 10.1212/WNL.0000000000003279

[48] Theodoroff SM, Griest SE, Folmer RL. Transcranial magnetic stimulation for tinnitus: Using the tinnitus functional index to predict benefit in a randomized controlled trial. Trials. 2017;**18**(1):64. DOI: 10.1186/s13063-017-1807-9

[49] Liang Z, Yang H, Cheng G, Huang L, Zhang T, Jia H. Repetitive transcranial magnetic stimulation on chronic tinnitus: A systematic review and meta-analysis. BMC Psychiatry. 2020;**20**(1):547. DOI: 10.1186/s12888-020-02947-9

[50] Soleimani R, Jalali MM, Hasandokht T. Therapeutic impact of repetitive transcranial magnetic stimulation (rTMS) on tinnitus: A systematic review and meta-analysis. European Archives of Oto-Rhino-Laryngology. 2016;**273**(7):1663-1675. DOI: 10.1007/s00405-015-3642-5

[51] Wang X et al. Effects of non-invasive brain stimulation on post-stroke spasticity: A systematic review and meta-analysis of randomized controlled trials. Brain Sciences. 2022;**12**(7):836. DOI: 10.3390/brainsci12070836

[52] Yang S et al. Effect of repetitive transcranial magnetic stimulation on pain management: A systematic narrative review. Frontiers in Neurology. 2020;**11**:114. DOI: 10.3389/fneur.2020.00114

[53] Attal N et al. Repetitive transcranial magnetic stimulation for neuropathic pain: A randomized multicentre

sham-controlled trial. Brain. 2021;**144**(11):3328-3339

[54] Wen X, Liu Z, Zhong L, Peng Y, Wang J, Liu H, et al. The effectiveness of repetitive transcranial magnetic stimulation for post-stroke dysphagia: A systematic review and meta-analysis. Frontiers in Human Neuroscience. 2022;**16**:841781. DOI: 10.3389/fnhum.2022.841781

[55] Xie YL, Wang S, Jia JM, Xie YH, Chen X, Qing W, et al. Transcranial magnetic stimulation for improving dysphagia after stroke: A meta-analysis of randomized controlled trials. Frontiers in Neuroscience. 2022;**16**:854219. DOI: 10.3389/fnins.2022.854219

[56] Müri RM, Cazzoli D, Nef T, Mosimann UP, Hopfner S, Nyffeler T. Non-invasive brain stimulation in neglect rehabilitation: An update. Frontiers in Human Neuroscience. 2013;7:248. DOI: 10.3389/fnhum.2013.00248

[57] Nahas E et al. Navigated perilesional transcranial magnetic stimulation can improve post-stroke visual field defect: A double-blind sham-controlled study. Restorative Neurology and Neuroscience. 2021;**39**(3):199-207

[58] Tsuboyama M et al. Review of transcranial magnetic stimulation in epilepsy. Clinical Therapeutics. 2020;**42**(7):1155-1168

[59] Manganotti P, Acler M, Masiero S, Del Felice A. TMS-evoked N100 responses as a prognostic factor in acute stroke. Functional Neurology. 2015;**30**(2):125-130. DOI: 10.11138/fneur/2015.30.2.125

[60] Voitenkov V, Klimkin A, Skripchenko N, et al. Diagnostic transcranial magnetic stimulation as a prognostic tool in children with acute transverse myelitis. Spinal Cord. 2016;**54**:226-228. DOI: 10.1038/sc.2015.129

[61] Jeltema HR, Ohlerth AK, de Wit A, Wagemakers M, Rofes A, Bastiaanse R, et al. Comparing navigated transcranial magnetic stimulation mapping and "gold standard" direct cortical stimulation mapping in neurosurgery: a systematic review. Neurosurgical Review. 2021;**44**(4):1903-1920. DOI: 10.1007/s10143-020-01397-x

[62] Picht T, Schmidt S, Brandt S, Frey D, Hannula H, Neuvonen T, et al. Preoperative functional mapping for rolandic brain tumor surgery: Comparison of navigated transcranial magnetic stimulation to direct cortical stimulation. Neurosurgery. 2011 Sep;**69**(3):581-588. DOI: 10.1227/NEU.0b013e3182181b89

[63] Haddad AF, Young JS, Berger MS, Tarapore PE. Preoperative applications of navigated transcranial magnetic stimulation. Frontiers in Neurology. 2021;**11**:628903. DOI: 10.3389/fneur.2020.628903

[64] Umana GE, Scalia G, Graziano F, Maugeri R, Alberio N, Barone F, et al. Navigated transcranial magnetic stimulation motor mapping usefulness in the surgical Management of Patients Affected by brain Tumors in eloquent areas: A systematic review and meta-analysis. Frontiers in Neurology. 2021;**12**:644198. DOI: 10.3389/fneur.2021.644198

[65] Sporns O, Tononi G, Kötter R. The human connectome: A structural description of the human brain. PLoS Computational Biology. 2005;**1**(4):e42. DOI: 10.1371/journal.pcbi.0010042

[66] Canali P. A role for TMS/EEG in neuropsychiatric disorders. Neurology

Psychiatry and Brain Research. 2014;**20**(2):37-40

[67] Cracco R, Amassian V, Maccabee P, Cracco J. Comparison of human transcallosal responses evoked by magnetic coil and electrical stimulation. Electroencephalography and Clinical Neurophysiology. 1989;**74**(6):417-424

[68] Farzan F, Vernet M, Shafi MM, Rotenberg A, Daskalakis ZJ, Pascual-Leone A. Characterizing and modulating brain circuitry through transcranial magnetic stimulation combined with electroencephalography. Front Neural Circuits. 2016;**10**:73. DOI: 10.3389/fncir.2016.00073

[69] Tremblay S, Rogasch NC, Premoli I, Blumberger DM, Casarotto S, Chen R, et al. Clinical utility and prospective of TMS-EEG. Clinical Neurophysiology. 2019;**130**(5):802-844. DOI: 10.1016/j.clinph.2019.01.001

Chapter 7

# Brain-Computer Interface: Use of Electroencephalogram in Neuro-Rehabilitation

*Ting Hin Adrian Hui*


## Abstract

Brain-computer interface is a technology that has been under enormous research in the last few decades. It uses brain signals by converting them into action to control the external environment. The focus of the future is the application of such technology in rehabilitating patients with physical disabilities. This chapter will mainly explore the use of EEG (electroencephalogram), a popular non-invasive method, on which the brain-computer interface is based. The process of signal extraction, selection and classification will be discussed. The challenges and techniques in communication and rehabilitation of people with motor impairment, along with the recent research study in this field, will be mentioned.


**Keywords:** brain-computer interface, electroencephalogram, neuro-rehabilitation, sensorimotor rhythm, evoked potential, motor imagery, hybrid, applications

## 1. Introduction

People with neuromuscular disorder suffer from various degrees of physical disabilities that limit them from interacting with the external world. Patients, who have developed stroke for instance resulting in paralysis and speech difficulties, would undergo training in traditional ways offered by physiotherapists, occupational and speech therapists. However, these trainings do require users' active participation to make rehabilitation effective. By performing such trainings, neuroplasticity can be induced through re-establishment of connections between the infarcted regions and other functional areas. As people do find traditional training to be tedious and slow, they are less motivated in engaging such therapy that results in suboptimal outcome. Besides, severely disabled patients who are tetraplegic or in lock-in state may not even benefit from the traditional rehabilitation at all. The invent of brain-computer interface (BCI) has opened up a new dimension of neurorehabilitation in this much needed population. BCI can as well improve neuroplasticity by using the signals from the brain and translating them into actions to control the external environment including robotic arms. Even just by thinking of a movement can exert similar control, a huge milestone for the severely disabled individuals to finally regain some control over their lives.

 

## 2. Overview of EEG-based BCI

Brain signals can be retrieved via invasive or non-invasive method. Invasive methods such as electrocorticography (ECoG) or intracortical point signal acquisition have the advantages of high temporal and spatial resolution with low artifact vulnerability. But with time, the signal quality and sensitivity would diminish. Non-invasive methods include electroencephalogram (EEG), magnetoencephalography (MEG), functional MRI (fMRI) and near-infrared spectroscopy (NIS) in general have high temporal resolution but with variable signal quality and spatial resolution [1].

### 2.1 Brain signals

EEG is our main focus in this chapter, and its use is widely popular due to low cost, low risk, portability and easy to set up. The downside would be poor signal quality and low spatial resolution. The signal can also be affected by external noise and artifact, along with mood and posture of the subjects. Upright posture can improve EEG quality due to stronger high-frequency content [2–4]. These brain signals can be classified as endogenous (spontaneous) and exogenous (evoked). The commonly used endogenous patterns are slow cortical potential (SCP) and sensorimotor rhythm (SMR); whereas, exogenous patterns are visual evoked potential (P300) and steady state visual evoked potentials (SSVEP) [1].

#### *2.1.1 Slow cortical potential*

Slow cortical potential arising from intracortical or thalamocortical region is projected to different cortical layers that harbor apical dendrites of pyramidal neurons. Firing from these neurons can generate motor or cognitive tasks. A negative voltage shift causes depolarization of the cortical network, while a positive voltage shift an inhibition (**Figure 1**). Intense training is required to control the shifting in the SCPs in order to perform basic tasks. As a result, these long training hours might hinder the popularity of the use of such brain signals [1].

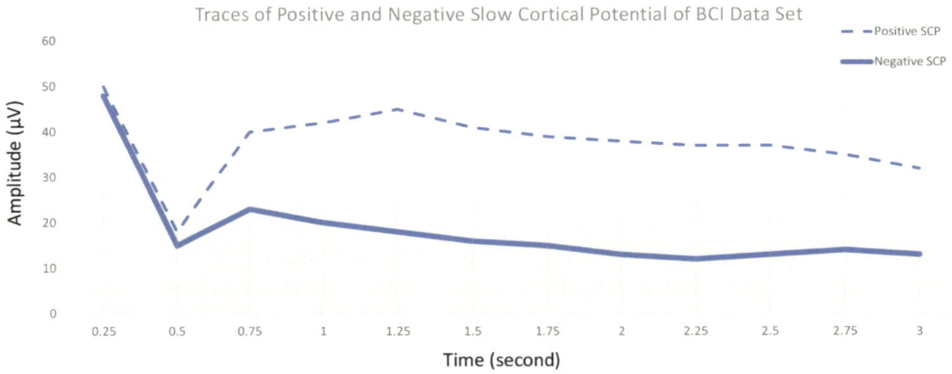


**Figure 1.**
*Mean traces of positive SCP and negative SCP of a BCI data set.*

### *2.1.2 Sensorimotor rhythm*

The sensorimotor rhythm arising from sensorimotor areas generates β (beta) and μ (mu) rhythm mainly used for specific voluntary regulations such as preparation, control and execution of motion. Merely the thought of a movement (**Figure 2**), without any external stimuli, can regulate the rhythm amplitudes in these central motor areas, which makes it appealing for users with severe motor disabilities. The change in the power of band frequency helps differentiate the type of mental tasks being carried out. A decrease in band frequency termed event-related desynchronization (ERD) occurs up to 2 seconds before the actual movement. Event-related synchronization (ERS) signifies an increase in the band frequency that occurs before the end of a movement. The classes of movement that can be identified through SMR are left hand movement, right hand movement, movement of the feet and movement of the tongue. But the movement between left and right foot and between particular fingers of one hand are indistinguishable due to their small representation in the cortical homunculus. Again, it requires intensive training and sufficient mental capacity and attention to generate this motor imagery-based EEG signals [1, 4].

### *2.1.3 Visual evoked potential*

Visual evoked potential (P300) occurs at 300 milliseconds after a triggering stimulus (**Figure 3**). Because the potential occurs with high consistency, this positive voltage peak has been used to mark an event. Although it requires less extensive

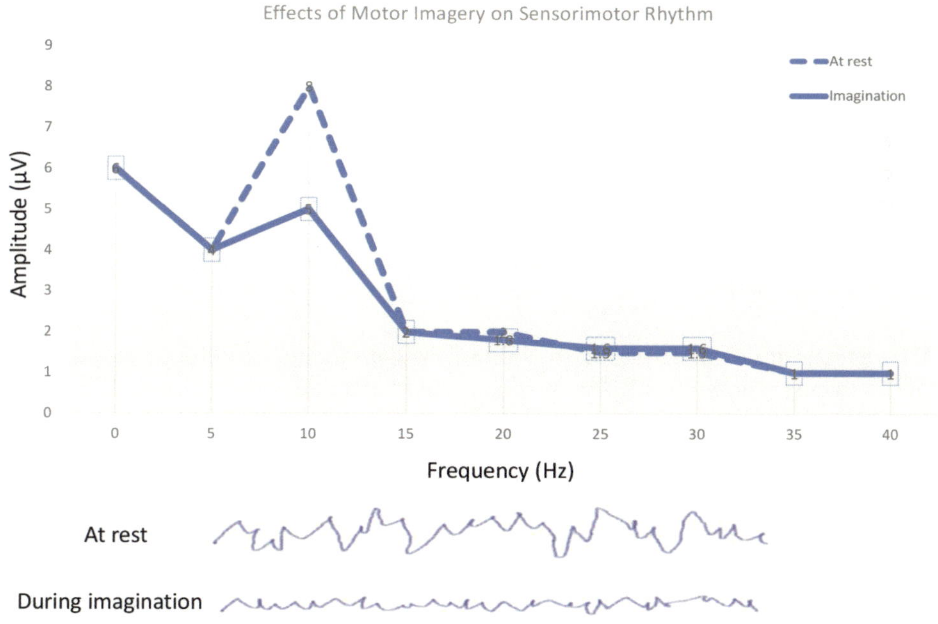


**Figure 2.**
*Effects of motor imagery on sensorimotor rhythm. On the top shows the frequency spectra during movement at rest (dashed line) and during imagination (solid line). During imagination, the amplitude of EEG tracing is attenuated as shown on the bottom.*

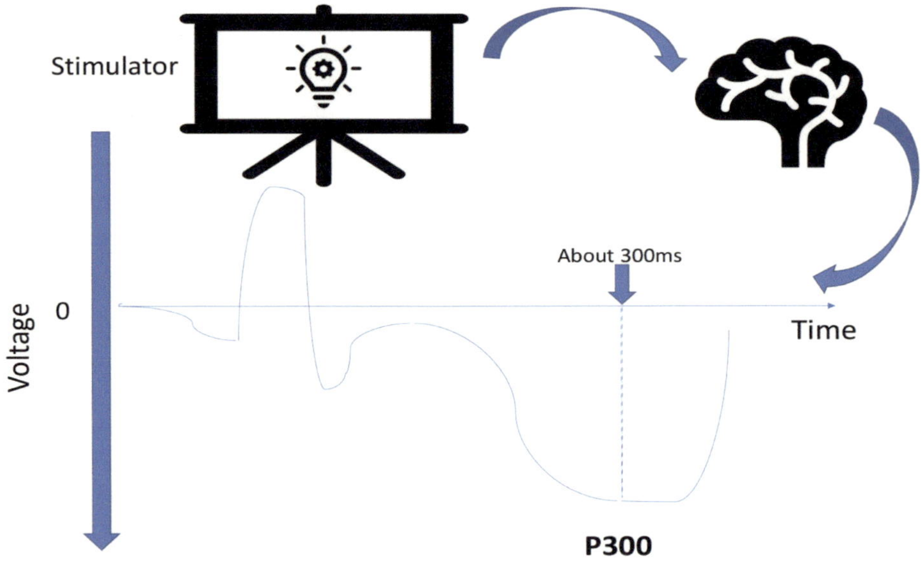


**Figure 3.**
*Visual evoked potential. This is initially stimulated by flashes on the screen, then captured by the brain producing a positive voltage potential occurs at 300 ms after the stimulus.*

training compared to SCP and SMR, the usefulness of P300 may be hampered by the severity of motor disabilities and degree of fatigue. Another visual evoked potential, called steady state visual evoked potentials (SSVEP), requires users' attention and the ability of visual fixation. The potentials are triggered by an oscillating stimulus at a fixed frequency, like a flashing letters or digits on a screen. That results in an increase in EEG activity, or SSVEP response, at the occipital area with the same frequency as the stimulus. However, the requirement of an intact oculomotor function and gaze fixation for a period of time has been challenging for some groups of patients. A study performed on amyotrophic lateral sclerosis (ALS) patients did not have much success due to their inability to control eye movement [1].

#### *2.1.4 Other brain signals*

Other techniques that are used to obtain EEG data include auditory evoked potential (a corresponding EEG pattern generated after an auditory stimulation), vibrotactile evoked potential (a corresponding EEG activity generated after physical vibrations at a particular frequency), imagined speech (imagination of words or sentences for evoking EEG signals), and error-related potential (an activity when a mismatch between the subject's intention and the output response from the BCI application is detected). One of the increasingly popular way to obtain EEG data is by analyzing EEG spectral changes to monitor users' drowsiness, attention, mental workload, emotions and other states of the mind [2]. This can become handy in detecting drivers' concentration at work, or in criminal cases when lie detector machine is employed.

### **2.2 Architecture of BCI system**

**Figure 4.**

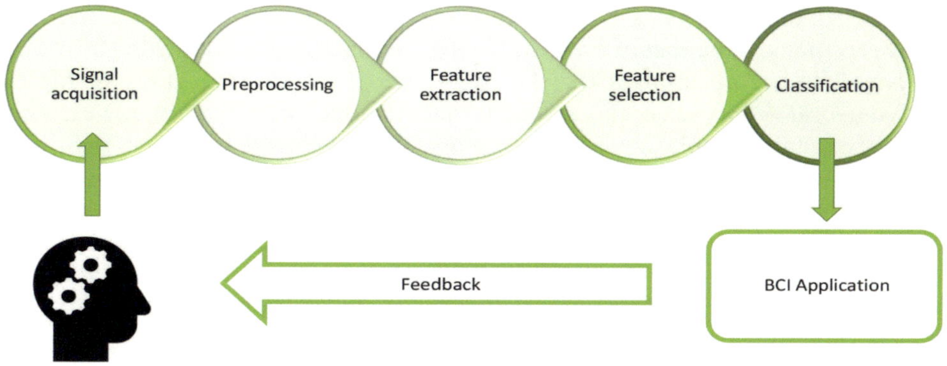


**Figure 4.**
*The architecture of a brain computer system consists of signal acquisition from the brain, pre-processing, feature extraction, feature selection, classification and eventually application to external devices that provides feedback to users.*

### *2.2.1 Data acquisition and pre-processing*

After the raw EEG data has been detected via the scalp electrodes, the data needs to remove any signals originated in areas other than the brain such as using the 60 Hz notch to clean the intervening frequency and the EMG activity before further analysis [1, 3]. After this pre-processing step, signal processing is performed using many different feature extraction techniques to identify specific brain signals that would later be translated to system commands [5].

### *2.2.2 Feature extraction*

There are numerous techniques that enable proper signals to be retrieved during feature extraction. We will not go into detail into each of the techniques, but some common ones are briefly discussed in this section. Time-domain and frequency-domain are two basic techniques often applied in studies. Using quaternions to represent objects within a three-dimensional space offers a better method to aid in extracting signals in time-domain analysis especially from motor imagery EEG. Fast Fourier transform theory and local characteristic-scale decomposition are approaches that are often utilized in frequency-domain analysis. In order to relate the frequency content to the temporal domain and vice versa, time-frequency domain analysis helps compensate each other's deficit in decomposing signals in a more dynamic fashion. Common spatial pattern (CSP) is advantageous in motor imagery EEG processing as it can extract particular information from a particular frequency band. Different modifications of CSP are available, and sub-band common spatial pattern offers a much better classification accuracy by initially filtering EEG at different sub-bands and then tabulating CSP features for each of the bands [4, 5].

### *2.2.3 Feature selection and classification*

The most common feature selection techniques include principal component analysis (PCA), filter bank selection and evolutionary algorithms. PCA helps to reduce dimensionality, while filter bank selection is specific for CSP extraction technique. Due to the high computational demands and large size feature set, evolutionary algorithm can further select a more appropriate feature by hybrid approach so to improve accuracy at the cost of time [4, 5]. For classification and modeling of the control system, linear discriminant analysis (LDA), support vector machines (SVM) and artificial neural networks (ANN) are the frequently used classifiers [6]. LDA is a linear classifier that is simple to use but it may not be good enough to process non-linear EEG data. SVM is a non-linear classifier that handles well with high dimensionality data; however, it takes more time for processing. ANN is another non-linear classifier that requires long handling time to process large computational data. It is known to be highly adaptive but also over-fitting; therefore, it may fail to predict future observations reliably [6]. Eventually, neurofeedback system relays back to the users so they can make modification in their brain patterns and improve the system.

## 3. Use of brain signals in reality

### 3.1 Slow cortical potential

Slow cortical potential as mentioned previously requires subjects to control the upward and downward shifting of polarity to select letters, words or pictograms. A system is developed to allow subjects to communicate through writing: first phase requires basic training for regulating own SCP amplitude by mental strategies either above or below a certain threshold to move the cursor at a specific space or time; and, the second phase requires selecting and rejecting letters by self-managing own SCP amplitudes to form words and phrases. One study also helps subjects to browse the Internet by training them to self-regulate SCP amplitudes to move up or down the cursor in order to select or discard a command [1].

### 3.2 P300 evoked potential

P300 is late positive evoked potential occurs after an external task-stimulus. The users are given different options of commands or stimuli, and the system needs to detect which stimuli can elicit P300 to exert its role on various systems like painting, spelling, web browsing and controlling of external devices [1]. Various BCI-controlled humanoid applications have been discussed in [6] like grasping a glass of water by robotics in ALS patients, controlling the navigation of a robot via telepresence. Using hybrid BCI by combining the brain signals (P300) and the biological feedback signals generated by some other parts of the body are also seen in executing the command [6]. The advantage of using P300 is its high accuracy. However, the performance is not consistently at a high level, mainly affected by the severity of the disease and the lack of motivation by repeatedly doing the same training routine [1].

### 3.3 Sensorimotor rhythm

Sensorimotor rhythm requires subjects to use mental strategies or motor imagery to enable motor execution (ME). For subjects who have motor disabilities, the thought of movement can suppress EEG rhythm leading to desynchronization, resulting in movement initiation. Motor imagery can enhance motor learning process by neuroplasticity [7, 8]. With both MI and ME derived from sensorimotor areas such as primary motor area, supplementary motor area and premotor cortex, SMR can be manipulated to help the disabled towards rehabilitation. The differences in the

BCI performance may be related to the number of folds and thickness of individuals' cortices which may have an impact on the functional networks. The emotional and mental processes such as fatigue, memory load, attention and reaction time, along with gender, age and lifestyle all contribute to the inter- and intra-variability in SMR-based BCI motor performance. Overall, subjects with high motor variability including force field adaptation, speed/trajectory, motivational factors and strong resting EEG amplitudes have a higher probability of achieving better BCI performance, hence better neuroplasticity and rehabilitation outcome [8].

Many BCI systems have been using SMR by means of spelling, cursor movement, and control of external devices for communication to the external world. Creating a virtual environment to work under, subjects are more motivated in controlling movement in this framework resulting in better performance with fewer runs of training [1].

## 4. BCI applications in rehabilitation

The applications for BCI systems in rehabilitation include motor neuroprosthetics, computer/machine interfaces, video games, speech and communication, meditation, and even art. The famous Hebbian theory, developed by Canadian psychologist Donald Hebb, described that with repeated stimulation of the postsynaptic neurons by presynaptic neurons, the efficacy of synaptic transmission would increase resulting in neuroplasticity. Besides, using the traditional rehabilitation therapy, BCI system can help "replace" and "restore" neurological functions by training patients to produce more reliable brain signals and to activate devices to assist movement [1, 3]. Patients with different cortical lesions may produce different oscillatory rhythm of neural activation [3].

### 4.1 Motor imagery

Evidence shows by using motor imagery, SMR can be trained to translate into commands to control and regulate voluntary activity. Just by imagining left or right hand movement, the right or left hemisphere respectively is activated, and the signals can be further processed and classified. To master MI-based BCI, subjects can undergo two approaches. The discrete trial, considered as tedious and lengthy, instructs them to perform cues within a timeframe while providing on-screen feedback on their results. On the other hand, continuous pursuit looks more promising as subjects are told to control a cursor in a moving icon on-screen. This provides a game-like approach so the subjects are more engaged with stronger brain signals being detected along with fewer training sessions required [9]. The challenges of using motor imagery are the requirement of a near-intact neurophysiological and psychological state of the users. This becomes a challenge to post-stroke patients with reduced in such mental and physical capacities [4].

### 4.2 Other paradigms

Other paradigms including spelling, induced emotions and facial-movement have also been tested to control wheelchair, prosthetic hand and robotic arm. Spelling the desired command has a higher accuracy but subjects may get fatigue with continuously spelling words to elicit the command. Inducing emotions is mentally demanding, while facial movement is more intuitive and easier to generate. Besides, this movement has lower illiteracy rates and higher accuracy rates. Merging different paradigms, for example combining traditional MI and facial movement, can increase the number of classes or control functions to overcome poor classification accuracy of MI system. Some studies require subjects to perform sequential movement to bring out a command. This increases the latency as each command takes up around 3 seconds. Therefore, more time is required for execution. No comparisons have been made so far between traditional and sequential command paradigm. Whether it is feasible to increase accuracy at the expense of increasing latency remains a question to be explored [9]. Combining another biosignal to increase the number of commands is called hybrid BCIs. To enhance the control of prosthetics or orthotics, merging EEG with EMG has become increasingly popular [9].

### 4.3 EEG: EMG application

Combined use of EEG and surface EMG in rehabilitative applications can control the effector's devices with a pathway starting from the cortical level down to the muscular level. EEG first explores the whole brain neuronal network, while EMG measures the train of motor unit action potentials that can help in motor planning with quantitative measurement in motor control abnormalities and muscular activation patterns. They combine with BCI or biofeedback methods to control external devices and guide rehabilitation. Using cortico-muscular coherence as signal analysis, it can "detect voluntary movements in spastic subjects, assess the effectiveness of rehabilitation strategies and serve as biomarker for motor recovery" [10]. As most of the experiments are done as pilot studies, more clinical trials are needed to evaluate the EEG–EMG applications [10].

### 4.4 Other studies

Voznenko [11] studies the design of wheelchair control that uses thoughts, voice or gestures to mobilize a wheelchair. The use of combined BCI-FES (functional electrical stimulation) as designed by Muller-Putz study [4] helps send impulses to the patients' paralyzed arm/leg by artificially contracting the muscles. Therefore, the patients can have a more authentic experience. In [4], a number of studies have also been mentioned. Muller-Putz and Pfurtschscheller's study [12] uses 4 flickering stimuli with each one representing a different function of the arm based on SSVEP system. Subjects can select a movement by looking at a particular stimulus. Elstob and Secco [13] uses motor imagery-BCI to control a prosthetic arm that consists of 5 different types of movement. Using virtual reality, BCI controlled robotic arms can potentially guide subjects' arm movement in post-stroke rehabilitation, like the system proposed by Luu [14]. It is suggested that brain activities be measured while users are moving on a treadmill, and then "provide visual feedback to the user on their movements through a virtual avatar" [4].

### 4.5 Modalities in rehabilitation

While research has mainly focused on motor rehabilitation, targets on improving tactile stimulus alone has been lacking. Sensory and motor cortices share the same somatic organization and are inseparable in improving and restoring function. Without sensory input, the rehabilitation of limbs would not be complete. Development of sensory-motor closed loop systems, or the bidirectional BCI, should improve the efficiency of rehabilitation in the future. In communication rehabilitation, patients with aphasia can regulate their evoked potentials (SCP, SMR, P300) to communicate by producing letters via a speller system. Limited by the severity of cognitive impairment in poststroke or neurodegenerative patients, they may not be benefited from BCI as some basic cognitive levels are required to understand and manipulate the application. Providing neurofeedback via motor imagery and P300 system may enhance the rehabilitative process in this group of populations. In sum, there is still a lot of research required in poststroke cognitive training [3].

## 5. Challenges and future direction

Finding the most effective technique for features extraction and selection has been a challenge as each technique has its own advantages and disadvantages. Besides, EEG itself is also highly non-linear and artifact-prone. Together, a low classification accuracy may result. Combining different classifiers or biosignals can improve this accuracy, but the training time to master the control is much prolonged which in turn affects the overall efficiency. Future studies using subjects with pathological disorders instead of healthy ones are encouraged so to increase the generalizability in the biomedical field. In terms of non-biomedical applications such as art, gaming and entertainment, this is a potential market that contributes to economic growth. However, developing a "dependable system with stable performance with different mental states" that can adapt to different environments is the main goal to gain its public acceptance in the next decade (**Table 1**) [4].

| Method | Description | Characteristics | Application in reality |
|---|---|---|---|
| Slow cortical potential (SCP) | • Endogenous signal to cause voltage shifting<br>• Negative voltage shift causing depolarization<br>• Positive voltage shift causing inhibition | • Requires intense training | Formation of words and phrases, browse internet by moving cursor to select or discard a command |
| Sensorimotor rhythm (SMR) | • Endogenous signal to generate β (beta) and μ (mu) rhythm<br>• Regulate rhythm amplitudes in central motor areas by motor imagery<br>• Change in power of band frequency to differentiate the type of mental tasks | • Requires intense training<br>• Requires mental capacity | Spelling, cursor movement, controlling external devices [11, 13] |
| Visual evoked potential | • Exogenous signal to generate a potential:<br>• at 300 ms after a triggering stimulus (P300)<br>• triggered by an oscillating stimulus at a fixed frequency (SSVEP) | • High consistency and accuracy<br>• Requires intact oculomotor function and gaze fixation<br>• Requires shorter training time | Painting, spelling, controlling external devices [12] |

**Table 1.**
*Comparative analysis of various methods used for recording features.*

## 6. Conclusion

We have discussed the basic architecture of BCI system using EEG as brain signals to control external devices in rehabilitation and communication. Exogenous and endogenous signals elicited by external stimuli and motor imagery respectively can enhance neuroplasticity and improve motor function. However, research on other modalities such as sensory and cognition are still at its primitive stage. Applications in the biomedical field are blooming but challenges in creating the best system that fits in all conditions still remain.

## Author details

Ting Hin Adrian Hui
United Christian Hospital, Hong Kong SAR, People's Republic of China

*Address all correspondence to: hth077@ha.org.hk

## References

[1] Lazarou I, Nikolopoulos S, Petrantonakis PC, Kompatsiaris I, Tsolaki M. EEG-based brain-computer interfaces for communication and rehabilitation of people with motor impairment: A novel approach of the 21st century. Frontiers in Human Neuroscience. 2018;**12**(14):1-18. DOI: 10.3389/fnhum.2018.00014

[2] Varbu K, Muhammad N, Muhammad Y. Past, present, future of EEG-based BCI applications. Sensors. 2022;**22**(3331):1-44. DOI: 10.3390/s22093331

[3] Yang S, Li R, Li H, Xu K, Shi Y, Wang Q, et al. Exploring the use of brain-computer interfaces in stroke neurorehabilitation. BioMed Research International. 2021;**2021**:1-11. DOI: 10.1155/2021/9967348

[4] Padfield N, Zabalza J, Zhao H, Masero V, Ren J. EEG-based brain-computer interfaces using motor-imagery: Techniques and challenges. Sensors. 2019;**19**(1423):1-34. DOI: 10.3390/s19061423

[5] Camargo-Vargas D, Callejas-Cuervo M, Mazzoleni S. Brain-computer interfaces systems for upper and lower limb rehabilitation: A systematic review. Sensors. 2021;**21**(4312):1-22. DOI: 10.3390/s21134312

[6] Chamola V, Vineet A, Nayyar A, Hossain E. Brain-computer interface-based humanoid control: A review. Sensors. 2020;**20**(3620):1-23. DOI: 10.3390/s20133620

[7] Nierhaus T, Vidaurre C, Sannelli C, Mueller KR, Villringer A. Immediate brain plasticity after one hour of brain-computer interface (BCI). The Journal of Physiology. 2021;**599**(9):2435-2451. DOI: 10.1113/JP278118

[8] Saha S, Baumert M. Intra- and inter-subject variability in EEG-based sensorimotor brain computer interface: A review. Frontiers in Computational Neuroscience. 2020;**13**(87):1-8. DOI: 10.3389/fncom.2019.00087

[9] Padfield N, Camilleri K, Camilleri T, Fabri S, Bugeja M. A comprehensive review of endogenous EEG-based BCIs for dynamic device control. Sensors. 2022;**22**(5802):1-36. DOI: 10.3390/s22155802

[10] Brambilla C, Pirovano I, Mira RM, Rizzo G, Scano A, Mastropietro A. Combined use of EMG and EEG techniques for neuromotor assessment in rehabilitative applications: A systematic review. Sensors. 2021;**21**(7014):1-25. DOI: 10.3390/s21217014

[11] Voznenko TI, Chepin EV, Urvanov GA. The control system based on extended BCI for a robotic wheelchair. Procedia Computer Science. 2018;**123**:522-527

[12] Müller-Putz GR, Pfurtscheller G. Control of an electrical prosthesis with an SSVEP-based BCI. IEEE Transactions on Biomedical Engineering. 2008;**55**:361-364

[13] Elstob D, Secco EL. A low cost EEG based BCI prosthetic using motor imagery. International Journal of Information Technology Convergence and Services. 2016;**6**(1):23-36

[14] Luu TP, Nakagome S, He Y, Contreras-Vidal JL. Real-time EEG-based brain-computer interface to a virtual avatar enhances cortical involvement in human treadmill walking. Scientific Reports. 2017;**7**(1):8895